Motility Consultation: Challenges in Gastrointestinal Motility in Everyday Clinical Practice

Guest Editor

EAMONN M.M. QUIGLEY, MD

GASTROENTEROLOGY CLINICS OF NORTH AMERICA

www.gastro.theclinics.com

December 2011 • Volume 40 • Number 4

SAUNDERS an imprint of ELSEVIER, Inc.

W.B. SAUNDERS COMPANY
A Division of Elsevier Inc.

Elsevier Inc. • 1600 John F. Kennedy Blvd., Suite 1800 • Philadelphia, Pennsylvania 19103-2899

http://www.theclinics.com

GASTROENTEROLOGY CLINICS OF NORTH AMERICA Volume 40, Number 4
December 2011 ISSN 0889-8553, ISBN-13: 978-1-4557-3986-8

Editor: Kerry Holland
Developmental Editor: Donald Mumford

Gastroenterology Clinics of North America (ISSN 0889-8553) is published quarterly by Elsevier Inc., 360 Park Avenue South, New York, NY 10010-1710. Months of issue are March, June, September, and December. Business and Editorial Offices: 1600 John F. Kennedy Blvd., Suite 1800, Philadelphia, PA 19103-2899. Customer Service Office: 6277 Sea Harbor Drive, Orlando, FL 32887-4800. Periodicals postage paid at New York, NY and additional mailing offices. Subscription prices are $305.00 per year (US individuals), $153.00 per year (US students), $488.00 per year (US institutions), $335.00 per year (Canadian individuals), $594.00 per year (Canadian institutions), $423.00 per year (international individuals), $211.00 per year (international students), and $594.00 per year (international institutions). Foreign air speed delivery is included in all *Clinics* subscription prices. All prices are subject to change without notice. **POSTMASTER:** Send address changes to *Gastroenterology Clinics of North America,* Elsevier Health Sciences Division, Subscription Customer Service, 3251 Riverport Lane, Maryland Heights, MO 63043. Telephone: 1-800-654-2452 (U.S. and Canada); 314-447-8871 (outside U.S. and Canada). Fax: 314-447-8029. E-mail: journalscustomerservice-usa@elsevier.com (for print support); journalsonlinesupport-usa@elsevier.com (for online support).

Reprints. For copies of 100 or more, of articles in this publication, please contact the Commercial Reprints Department, Elsevier Inc., 360 Part Avenue South, New York, New York 10010-1710. Tel. (212) 633-3813, Fax: (212) 462-1935, E-mail: reprints@elsevier.com.

Gastroenterology Clinics of North America is also published in Italian by Il Pensiero Scientifico Editore, Rome, Italy; and in Portuguese by Interlivros Edicoes Ltda., Rua Commandante Coelho 1085, 21250 Cordovil, Rio de Janeiro, Brazil.

Gastroenterology Clinics of North America is covered in *MEDLINE/PubMed (Index Medicus), Excerpta Medica, Current Contents/Clinical Medicine, Science Citation Index, ISI/BIOMED,* and *BIOSIS.*

Printed and bound by CPI Group (UK) Ltd, Croydon, CR0 4YY

Transferred to Digital Print 2011

Contributors

GUEST EDITOR

EAMONN M.M. QUIGLEY, MD, FRCP, FACP, FACG, FRCPI
Professor of Medicine and Human Physiology, Department of Medicine, Alimentary Pharmabiotic Centre, University College Cork, Cork, Ireland

AUTHORS

AURELIEN AMIOT, MD
Hôpital Beaujon, Service Gastreonterologie, MICI et Assistance Nutritive Aproved Center for HPN and Intestinal Failure, Université Paris VII, Clichy, France

GIOVANNI BARBARA, MD
Associate Professor of Medicine, Department of Clinical Medicine, University of Bologna, St. Orsola-Malpighi Hospital; Neurogastrenterology and Motility Laboratory, University of Bologna, Bologna, Italy

ADIL E. BHARUCHA, MBBS, MD
Clinical Enteric Neurosciences Translational and Epidemiological Research Program, Division of Gastroenterology and Hepatology, Mayo Clinic and Mayo Foundation, Rochester, Minnesota

R. BISSCHOPS, MD, PhD
Department of Gastroenterology, University Hospital of Leuven and Catholic University of Leuven, Leuven, Belgium

G.E. BOECKXSTAENS, MD, PhD
Department of Gastroenterology, Translational Research Center for Gastrointestinal Disorders (TARGID), University Hospital of Leuven and Catholic University of Leuven, Leuven, Belgium

MARIANNE J. CHAPMAN, BMBS, PhD, FCICM
Associate Professor, Department of Critical Care Services, Royal Adelaide Hospital; Discipline of Acute Care Medicine, School of Medicine, University of Adelaide, Adelaide, South Australia, Australia

ROSANNA F. COGLIANDRO, MD, PhD
Assistant Professor of Medicine, Department of Clinical Medicine, University of Bologna, St. Orsola-Malpighi Hospital; Neurogastrenterology and Motility Laboratory, University of Bologna, Bologna, Italy

ROBERTO CORINALDESI, MD
Professor of Medicine and Head of the Department of Clinical Medicine, University of Bologna, St. Orsola-Malpighi Hospital; Neurogastrenterology and Motility Laboratory, University of Bologna, Bologna, Italy

ADAM M. DEANE, MBBS, FRACP, FCICM
Staff Specialist and Senior Lecturer, Department of Critical Care Services, Royal Adelaide Hospital; Discipline of Acute Care Medicine, School of Medicine, University of Adelaide, Adelaide, South Australia, Australia

JOHN K. DIBAISE, MD
Professor of Medicine, Division of Gastroenterology and Hepatology, Mayo Clinic, Scottsdale, Arizona

ROBERTO DE GIORGIO, MD, PhD
Associate Professor of Medicine, Department of Clinical Medicine, University of Bologna, St. Orsola-Malpighi Hospital; Neurogastrenterology and Motility Laboratory, University of Bologna, Bologna, Italy

ZAID HEETUN, MB, MRCPI
Specialist Registrar in Internal Medicine and Gastroenterology, Department of Medicine, Alimentary Pharmabiotic Centre, University College Cork, Cork, Ireland

FRANCISCA JOLY, MD, PhD
Hôpital Beaujon, Service Gastreonterologie, MICI et Assistance Nutritive Aproved Center for HPN and Intestinal Failure, Université Paris VII, Clichy, France

PETER J. KAHRILAS, MD, AGAF
Professor, Department of Medicine, Feinberg School of Medicine, Northwestern University, Chicago, Illinois

CHARLES H. KNOWLES, BChir, PhD, FRCS
Clinical Professor of Surgical Research, Academic Surgical Unit, Centre for Digestive Diseases, Blizard Institute, Barts and the London School of Medicine and Dentistry, Queen Mary University London, London, United Kingdom

GREGER LINDBERG, MD, PhD
Karolinska Institutet, Department of Medicine, Karolinska University Hospital, Stockholm, Sweden

JOANNE E. MARTIN, PhD, FRCPath
Professor of Pathology, Pathology Group, Blizard Institute, Barts and the London, School of Medicine and Dentistry, Queen Mary University London, London, United Kingdom

MASSIMO MARTINELLI, MD
Medical Doctor, Department of Pediatrics, University of Naples "Federico II," Naples, Italy.

BERNARD MESSING, MD, PhD
Hôpital Beaujon, Service Gastreonterologie, MICI et Assistance Nutritive Aproved Center for HPN and Intestinal Failure, Université Paris VII, Clichy, France

NAM Q. NGUYEN, MBBS (Hons), PhD, FRACP
Staff Specialist and Senior Lecturer, Department of Gastroenterology and Hepatology, Royal Adelaide Hospital; Discipline of Medicine, School of Medicine, University of Adelaide, Adelaide, South Australia, Australia

SEAMUS O'MAHONY, MD, FRCP
Consultant Physician and Gastroenterologist, Gastroenterology, Cork University Hospital, Cork, Ireland

EAMONN M.M. QUIGLEY, MD, FRCP, FACP, FACG, FRCPI
Professor of Medicine and Human Physiology, Department of Medicine, Alimentary Pharmabiotic Centre, University College Cork, Cork, Ireland

W.O. ROHOF, MD
Department of Gastroenterology and Hepatology, Academic Medical Center, Amsterdam, The Netherlands

SABINE ROMAN, MD, PhD
Visiting Scholar, Department of Medicine, Feinberg School of Medicine, Northwestern University, Chicago, Illinois; Associate Professor, Digestive Physiology, Claude Bernard Lyon I University and Hospices Civils de Lyon, Lyon, France

ANNAMARIA STAIANO, MD
Associate Professor, Department of Pediatrics, University of Naples "Federico II," Naples, Italy

VINCENZO STANGHELLINI, MD
Professor of Medicine, Department of Clinical Medicine, University of Bologna, St. Orsola-Malpighi Hospital; Neurogastrenterology and Motility Laboratory, University of Bologna, Bologna, Italy

J. TACK, MD, PhD
Department of Gastroenterology, Translational Research Center for Gastrointestinal Disorders (TARGID), University Hospital of Leuven and Catholic University of Leuven, Leuven, Belgium

HANS TÖRNBLOM, MD, PhD
Karolinska Institutet, Department of Medicine, Karolinska University Hospital, Stockholm, Sweden

Contents

Preface: The Motility Consultation **xiii**

Eamonn M.M. Quigley

Erratum **xv**

Enteric Neuromuscular Pathology Update **695**

Charles H. Knowles and Joanne E. Martin

Clinically, study of the neuromuscular pathology of digestive motility disorders equates with study and histologic examination of biopsied or resected full-thickness human gastrointestinal tissues. This article covers several general principles and problems of diagnosis in this field from the perspective of methodological and interpretative variability. It then addresses the main current indications for histologic examination of tissues from patients with suspected enteric neuromuscular disease on the basis of clinically defined primary and secondary digestive motility disorders. It considers findings in achalasia, gastroparesis, intestinal pseudo-obstruction, enteric dysmotility, slow-transit constipation, and megacolon, thereby highlighting recent important findings and ongoing challenges.

A 21st Century Look at the Spectrum of Gastrointestinal Motility Disorders. What is Dysmotility; What is Functional? **715**

Hans Törnblom and Greger Lindberg

Physiology-based diagnosis of gastrointestinal motility disorders has a substantial overlap with symptom-based diagnosis. Neither symptomatic treatment nor therapy aimed at restoring normal physiology has had much success. However, the addition of physiology parameters to the evaluation of therapeutic interventions aimed at symptom reduction in functional gastrointestinal disorders can possibly facilitate the identification of subgroups with a higher probability of treatment success. In the ideal situation, the development of measurement methods with better availability and standardization will help us to merge physiology and symptoms regarding both diagnosis and treatment evaluation.

Gastrointestinal Dysmotility: Clinical Consequences and Management of the Critically Ill Patient **725**

Marianne J. Chapman, Nam Q. Nguyen, and Adam M. Deane

Abnormal gastrointestinal motility is a common feature of critical illness and results in a number of clinical problems that can complicate the management of patients in the intensive care unit. In this review the authors outline and describe the abnormalities in motility, their clinical sequelae, and the priorities of management. Reduced lower gastroesophageal sphincter pressures can result in esophageal reflux, slow gastric emptying leads to reduced success of gastric feeding, and impaired small intestinal motility may be associated with reduced nutrient absorption. Targeted treatment includes the administration of prokinetic agents and the delivery of nutrition directly into the small intestine.

Motility Disorders in the Patient with Neurologic Disease **741**

Eamonn M.M. Quigley, Seamus O'Mahony, and Zaid Heetun

As populations age, neurologic disease increases, and consultations relating to gastrointestinal motility problems become more common. Striated muscle under somatic control at either ends of the gastrointestinal tract, together with the modulatory effects of the autonomic nervous system on gut function and the many biological similarities between the enteric and central nervous systems, set the stage for disorders of gut motor and sensory function in neurologic disease. Oropharyngeal dysphagia, gastroparesis, constipation, and fecal incontinence are common in these patients. Assessment and management present several clinical and ethical problems and are best achieved with a dedicated and skilled multidisciplinary team.

Motility Problems in the Intellectually Challenged Child, Adolescent, and Young Adult **765**

Massimo Martinelli and Annamaria Staiano

Gastrointestinal (GI) motility problems represent an important cause of morbidity and sometimes mortality in patients affected by developmental disorders. This article describes motility disorders in Down syndrome, cerebral palsy, familial dysautonomia, and Williams syndrome. These problems do not often receive appropriate attention, either because priority is given to other medical aspects of the disorder, or because of the inability of affected children to communicate their symptoms. A better approach to the diagnosis and treatment of GI disorders is required to improve quality of life and minimize morbidity and mortality among patients with developmental disorders.

Paraneoplastic Gastrointestinal Dysmotility: When to Consider and How to Diagnose **777**

John K. DiBaise

There is a well-recognized association between malignant tumors and paraneoplastic gastrointestinal (GI) dysmotility. The detection of onconeural antibodies in a patient with suspected paraneoplastic GI dysmotility based on high-risk clinical features appears to be the most valuable diagnostic test and should prompt an aggressive search for an occult neoplasm. Management of paraneoplastic GI dysmotility syndromes is generally centered on treatment of the underlying malignancy along with conventional care of the GI dysmotility, nutritional support, and, occasionally, immunotherapy. Although rare, clinicians must be aware of the association between malignancy and GI dysmotility so that they know when to investigate for an underlying malignancy.

Chronic Intestinal Pseudo-Obstruction: Clinical Features, Diagnosis, and Therapy **787**

Roberto De Giorgio, Rosanna F. Cogliandro, Giovanni Barbara, Roberto Corinaldesi, and Vincenzo Stanghellini

Chronic intestinal pseudo-obstruction (CIPO) is a rare and severe condition characterized by a marked impairment of gut propulsive motility mimicking a mechanical obstruction in the absence of any demonstrable mechanical cause of luminal constriction of the gastrointestinal tract. Abnormalities of the enteric neuromuscular control systems may account for the gut dysmotility observed in CIPO. Patients with CIPO usually experience disabling symptoms and potentially life-threatening complications which may go unrecognized. Nutritional support is often required and is a cornerstone of the management of patients with CIPO. Medical and surgical therapeutic options are generally unsatisfactory and long-term outcome is poor in most cases.

Postoperative Problems 2011: Fundoplication and Obesity Surgery **809**

W.O. Rohof, R. Bisschops, J. Tack, and G.E. Boeckxstaens

Although the surgical treatment of both gastroesophageal reflux disease (GERD) and obesity is very successful, these procedures have a significant impact on the physiology and function of the proximal gastrointestinal tract. With the increasing prevalence of both GERD and obesity, more and more patients present at the motility outpatient clinic with symptoms related to surgical interventions for these medical problems. In this review, the authors describe the main complications following antireflux surgery: dysphagia, gas bloat syndrome, recurrent (persistent) GERD symptoms, and dyspeptic symptoms. The most common motility-related complications of obesity surgery are dumping syndrome and esophageal dysmotility.

Challenges in the Swallowing Mechanism: Nonobstructive Dysphagia in the Era of High-Resolution Manometry and Impedance **823**

Sabine Roman and Peter J. Kahrilas

Esophageal high-resolution manometry (HRM) improves the management of patients with nonobstructive dysphagia. It has increased the diagnostic yield for detecting achalasia and defined three clinically relevant achalasia subtypes. Esophagogastric junction (EGJ) outflow obstruction, defined as an impaired EGJ relaxation in association with some preserved peristalsis, might also represent an achalasia variant in some cases. Using the concept of distal latency, the criteria for defining distal esophageal spasm, have been revised as the occurrence of premature distal contractions. Finally, the combination of HRM and impedance monitoring allows for a functional definition of weak peristalsis associated with incomplete bolus transit.

Difficult Defecation: Difficult Problem Assessment and Management; What Really Helps? **837**

Adil E. Bharucha

A subset of patients with chronic constipation, up to 50% at tertiary centers, have difficult defecation, which can be suspected by clinical features and confirmed by anorectal tests. Symptoms of difficult defecation (ie, defecatory disorders) may occur in isolation or in association with symptoms of irritable bowel syndrome (IBS). Patients with defecatory disorders may have normal or slow colonic transit. Defecatory disorders should be recognized early because pelvic floor retraining by biofeedback therapy is superior to laxatives for management.

Nutritional Support in the Severely Compromised Motility Patient: When and How? **845**

Francisca Joly, Aurelien Amiot, and Bernard Messing

The management of chronic intestinal pseudo-obstruction (CIPO) remains difficult and requires a multidisciplinary approach. In adult patients with CIPO on home parenteral nutrition (HPN), the 10-year survival rate was 68%. Long-term HPN dependence does not seem to be associated with a significant increase in mortality and morbidity. HPN could be a safe and efficient approach to the management of intestinal failure caused by CIPO, with restoring oral intake and lowering hospitalization frequency as major goals of treatment.

Index **853**

FORTHCOMING ISSUES

March 2012
Modern Management of Benign and Malignant Pancreatic Disease
Jacques Van Dam, MD, PhD,
Guest Editor

June 2012
Chronic Diarrhea
Heinz Hammer, MD,
Guest Editor

September 2012
Evaluation of Inflammatory Bowel Disease
Samir Shah, MD, Edward Feller, MD, and Adam Harris, MD, *Guest Editors*

RECENT ISSUES

September 2011
Hepatology Update: Current Management and New Therapies
David A. Sass, MD, *Guest Editor*

June 2011
Women's Issues in Gastroenterology
Asyia Ahmad, MD, MPH,
and Barbara B. Frank, MD,
Guest Editors

March 2011
Irritable Bowel Syndrome
William D. Chey, MD,
Guest Editor

ISSUES OF RELATED INTEREST

Gastrointestinal Endoscopy Clinics of North America, January 2011 (Volume 21, Issue 1)
Advances in the Diagnosis and Management of Barrett's Esophagus
Irving Waxman, MD, FASGE, *Guest Editor*

Preface
The Motility Consultation

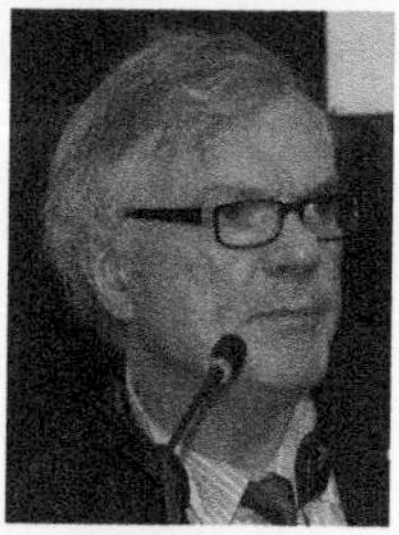

Eamonn M.M. Quigley, MD, FRCP, FRCPI
Guest Editor

The study of gastrointestinal motility and those disorders that result from its disordered function has, for far too long, been a much neglected component of every gastroenterology curriculum. Clinicians are "put off" by discussions of motility that, in their view, appear to focus on details of gut electrophysiology, neurotransmitter function, and enteric neural morphology, while, in "real life," disorders apparently resulting from pathology or dysfunction of enteric nerve and muscle and/or of the factors that control them go ignored. This neglect has been unfortunate given rapid progress in our understanding of the molecular and morphological basis of motor activity and of the physiology and basic pharmacology of motility, the advent of new approaches to the clinical assessment of disordered function, and an ever-increasing appreciation of the true frequency and clinical importance of dysmotility, be it in relation to a primary disorder of muscle or nerve, in the patient with cancer, in the context of a systemic or neurological disorder, or a consequence of a variety of therapeutic interventions. The clinician's despair when confronted by a "motility problem" has not been helped by a very poor record in translating progress in the laboratory into useful therapies at the bedside.

This issue of *Gastroenterology Clinics of North America* attempts to redress this deficit by taking a very different approach to gastrointestinal motility and viewing it primarily from a clinical, rather than physiological or pathophysiological, perspective. Individual articles are framed, therefore, in a clinical context: the intensive care unit, the patient with neurological disease, the postoperative patient, for example. The clinical usefulness of new technologies is illustrated by the impact of high-resolution manometry on the classification of esophageal motor disorders and of various imaging modalities on the assessment of difficult defecation. To bridge the gap between bench and bedside, progress in our understanding of the basic pathology of motility disorders is emphasized in the opening article and the clinical relevance of these classifications developed further by Greger Lindberg.

Some therapeutic optimism is also provided by a critical review of the indications for and optimal mode of delivery of nutritional support and new therapeutic

Gastroenterol Clin N Am 40 (2011) xiii–xiv
doi:10.1016/j.gtc.2011.10.001

approaches dealt with in each of the clinical scenario articles. We hope that this issue will help the clinician to recognize dysmotility in contexts where he or she would not previously had considered its role, optimally assess the issue, and develop a therapeutic strategy that will be of most benefit to the patient.

Eamonn M.M. Quigley, MD, FRCP, FRCPI
Department of Medicine
Alimentary Pharmabiotic Centre
University College Cork
Cork, Ireland

E-mail address:
e.quigley@ucc.ie

Erratum

Please note a correction is necessary in the article, "Hepatorenal Syndrome: Do the Vasoconstrictors Work?" by Drs Wesley Leung and Florence Wong, which published in the September 2011 issue of *Gastroenterology Clinics of North America* (40:3, pp 581–598). Following are the corrected source lines for Figures 2 and 3:

Figure 2a: From Sanyal AJ, Boyer T, Garcia-Tsao G, et al. A randomized, prospective, double-blind, placebo-controlled trial of terlipressin for type 1 hepatorenal syndrome. Gastroenterology 2008;134:1360–8; with permission.

Figure 2b: From Martín-Llahí M, Pépin MN, Guevara M, et al. Terlipressin and albumin vs albumin in patients with cirrhosis and hepatorenal syndrome: a randomized study. Gastroenterology 2008;134:1352–9; with permission.

Figure 3: From Sharma P, Kumar A, Shrama BC et al. An open label, pilot, randomized controlled trial of noradrenaline versus terlipressin in the treatment of type 1 hepatorenal syndrome and predictors of response. Am J Gastroenterol 2008;103:1689–97; with permission.

Gastroenterol Clin N Am 40 (2011) xv
doi:10.1016/j.gtc.2011.10.002
0889-8553/11/$ – see front matter

Enteric Neuromuscular Pathology Update

Charles H. Knowles, BChir, PhD, FRCS[a,*],
Joanne E. Martin, PhD, FRCPath[b]

KEYWORDS

- Gastrointestinal neuromuscular disease
- Intestinal pseudo-obstruction • Gastroparesis • Constipation
- Enteric neuropathy • Enteric myopathy

This issue of *Gastroenterology Clinics of North America* is focused on challenges faced in everyday clinical practice. Thus rather than reviewing the evolving research literature that details the many experimental models of enteric neuromuscular disease, this article considers the problems faced by the practicing pathologist, who, faced with a single tight-focus histologic "snapshot" of surgically derived tissue must decide whether disease of nerve, smooth muscle, or interstitial cells of Cajal (ICC) are present. This raises several technical and interpretational challenges (**Box 1**). Several of these points have been addressed in recent publications of an International Working Group (IWG) for GI neuromuscular pathology,[1–3] and much of this review draws on the IWG's important contributions to consensus in this field.

AVAILABILITY OF FULL-THICKNESS TISSUE

It is evident that diagnoses that depend on histologic examination of nerve, muscle, and ICC cannot be made using standard endoscopic biopsies. Thus in the main, tissues studied must be derived from full-thickness, or near full-thickness, biopsies taken with deliberate diagnostic intent or alternatively as the byproduct of emergency or planned surgical interventions. On this basis, tissues may take the form of deep seromuscular or full-thickness biopsies or resection specimens. The role of suction rectal biopsies in the management of Hirschsprung disease (HSCR) is well established and is not discussed further here. Regrettably, there are few other well

Prof. J.E. Martin is supported by the BBSRC and the Pseudo-obstruction Research Trust.
Mr. Charles H. Knowles is funded by the Higher Education Funding Council for England (H.E.F.C.E).

[a] Academic Surgical Unit, Centre for Digestive Diseases, Blizard Institute, Barts and the London School of Medicine and Dentistry, Queen Mary University London, UK
[b] Pathology Group, Blizard Institute, Barts and the London School of Medicine and Dentistry, Queen Mary University London, London, UK
* Corresponding author. Academic Surgical Unit, Centre for Digestive Diseases, 3rd Floor Alexandra Wing, Royal London Hospital, Whitechapel, London E1 1BB, UK.
E-mail address: c.h.knowles@qmul.ac.uk

Gastroenterol Clin N Am 40 (2011) 695–713
doi:10.1016/j.gtc.2011.09.007
0889-8553/11/$ – see front matter

Box 1
Histopathologic challenges in the diagnosis of enteric neuromuscular disease

Technical

1. Availability of adequate full-thickness tissue for study
2. Standardization of preparative (suitable fixation and orientation) and staining methods
3. Limitations on availability of more complex methods

Interpretational

4. Availability of normative human data
5. Clear definition of abnormality (in the individual)
6. Understanding of relationship of abnormality to observed clinical phenotype
7. Impact on patient management or prognosis

documented instances in which biopsy diagnoses clearly alter clinical care. Thus, although there are times that a bowel segment is discarded at the time of surgery and can be legitimately processed without additional risk to the patient, incidental biopsy at the time of other surgeries or as a planned procedure is more difficult to justify. Nevertheless, there is increasing evidence[4,5] and agreement[2] that minimally invasive (laparoscopic) biopsy techniques add little risk, which may be acceptable, in the context of improving the situation for the patient with severe symptoms in whom structural lesions detectable using radiologic and endoscopic techniques are absent. There is, however, no certainty that structural evidence of disease should be sought using full-thickness biopsy in all patients with otherwise unexplained abnormalities of gastrointestinal (GI) motor activity. Further, limitation on number (usually one) and size of biopsy inevitably leads to the possibility of sampling error in patchy diseases such as focal plexitis or leiomyositis.[6]

STANDARDIZATION OF PREPARATIVE AND STAINING METHODS

The main aim of the first IWG guideline, published in 2009,[2] was to evaluate the literature and bring together expert opinion to set acceptable standards of practice for the general pathologist in regard to procurement and preparation of tissue for study, methods of sectioning, and evaluation by routine and other techniques. The IWG noted that extraordinary variability existed in histopathologic techniques used for the study of tissues from patients with suspected GI neuromuscular pathology with wide differences in methodologies and expertise continuing to confound the significance and reliability of a variety of reported histopathologic changes in terms of clear delineation from normality. This was highlighted by a prior survey of practice in which 86 out of 130 European and U.S. histopathology laboratories processed tissue for suspected GI neuromuscular pathology, but only 33 performed more than a single hematoxylin and eosin (H&E) section. Of those that did more specialized tests, none did exactly the same tests.[7] Methodological issues are discussed for specific histopathologic findings in the text that follows.

LIMITATIONS ON AVAILABILITY OF MORE COMPLEX METHODS

The IWG was cognizant of the problems faced by general pathologists who receive specimens very infrequently and who may not have resources at their disposal to perform methods that require inordinate effort or specialized equipment. Thus, many techniques employed in the research literature are not relevant to challenges in everyday practice. These include the use of thick sections, multiple immunolabeling, and fluorescence and confocal microscopic or ultrastructural techniques. The IWG collated several referral recommendations for equivocal diagnoses that might benefit from further, more complex, studies at an index or specialist laboratory. Where results from these techniques may become relevant to future practice they have been included in this review but indicated as such.

AVAILABILITY OF NORMATIVE HUMAN DATA

The definition of disease (see the section that follows) is dependent on a clear concept of what constitutes normality, which is a particular problem when diagnoses depend on subtle qualitative or quantitative findings. This is exemplified by neuropathy or loss of ganglion cells wherein lack of adequate control data for elements of the human enteric nervous system (neuronal cell bodies, glial cells, and nerve fibres) led the IWG to systematically review 40 studies using techniques that could be deemed applicable to the practicing pathologist. The results revealed a disappointing lack of concordance between observations of different investigators, resulting in data insufficient to produce robust normal ranges.[3] This diversity further affirms the need to standardize the way pathologists collect, process, and quantitate neuronal and glial elements and to make a diagnosis only within the limits of confidence in the sample size. For instance, in the only available controlled study analyzing myenteric neuron counts in the whole circumference of the infant rectum, reliable estimates of the actual neuronal density required at least five full-circumference sections.[8]

CLEAR DEFINITION OF ABNORMALITY (IN THE INDIVIDUAL)

The diagnosis of disease in an individual is very different from establishing that significant differences exist in a particular quantitative finding between groups of patients and controls. The latter gives valuable information on the possible biology of disease but does not necessarily help define the cutoff for diagnosis for the pathologist facing a histologic section. This problem does not occur in categorical decisions based on binary qualitative observations, for example, neurons present or absent, muscle vacuolation and fibrosis present or absent. Unfortunately, such diagnoses are limited, in the most part, to infantile phenotypes of which most, for example, HSCR and hollow visceral myopathy, are rare or readily suspected on clinical/radiologic grounds. The situation is quite different in the more common diagnostic conundrum—that of the adult with chronic disordered motility and pain. Here, many patients have subtle neuropathic findings[4,5] and the situation is akin to that of small-bowel manometry, in which several studies attest to quantitative abnormalities of the migrating motor complex between patient and control cohorts but normal ranges are so wide that a firm diagnosis in an individual based on whether they fall within or without the normal range is still very difficult.[9] Diagnoses with established definitions that met consensus[1] are listed in **Table 1**; diagnostic criteria for these are shown in **Table 2**.

UNDERSTANDING THE RELATIONSHIP OF ABNORMALITY TO OBSERVED CLINICAL PHENOTYPE

Having decided that an adequately prepared and stained representative histopathologic section is abnormal, it is quite a different question as to whether the "validated" histopathologic diagnosis has a specific or causal relationship with the clinical

Table 1
The London classification of GI neuromuscular pathology

Neuropathies	**Subclassification**
1.1 Absent neurons	1.1.1 Aganglionosis
1.2 Decreased numbers of neurons	1.2.1 Hypoganglionosis
1.3 Increased numbers of neurons	1.3.1 Ganglioneuromatosis
	1.3.2 IND, type B
1.4 Degenerative neuropathy	
1.5 Inflammatory neuropathies	1.5.1 Lymphocytic ganglionitis
	1.5.2 Eosinophilic ganglionitis
1.6 Abnormal content in neurons	1.6.1 Intraneuronal nuclear inclusions
	1.6.2 Megamitochondria
1.7 Abnormal neurochemical coding	
1.8 Relative immaturity of neurons	
1.9 Abnormal enteric glia	1.9.1 Increased numbers of enteric glia
Myopathies	
2.1 Muscularis propria malformations	
2.2 Muscle cell degeneration	2.2.1 Degenerative leiomyopathy
	2.2.2 Inflammatory leiomyopathy
	2.2.2.1 Lymphocytic leiomyositis
	2.2.2.2 Eosinophilic leiomyositis
2.3 Muscle hyperplasia/hypertrophy	2.3.1 Muscularis mucosae hyperplasia
2.4 Abnormal content in myocytes	2.4.1 Filament protein abnormalities
	2.4.1.1 Alpha-actin myopathy
	2.4.1.2 Desmin myopathy
	2.4.2 Inclusion bodies
	2.4.2.1 Polyglucosan bodies
	2.4.2.2 Amphophilic
	2.4.2.3 Megamitochondria
2.5 Abnormal supportive tissue	2.5.1 Atrophic desmosis
Interstitial cell of Cajal abnormalities (enteric mesenchymopathy)	
3.1 Abnormal ICC networks	

Reproduced from Knowles CH, De Giorgio R, Kapur RP, et al. The London Classification of gastrointestinal neuromuscular pathology: report on behalf of the Gastro 2009 International Working Group. Gut 2010;59(7):882–7; *with permission.*

indication for biopsy. A second consensus process was undertaken by the IWG to address this issue[1] with development of a matrix between defined histopathologic phenotypes (from the London Classification) and recognized clinical entities using the development of two "diagnostic grades" (*etiologic* or *morphologic* associated) to indicate strength of relationship. Whereas criteria for making any association were the retrieval of two peer-reviewed publications from different institutions, the decision between etiologic and morphologic was decided by consensus, which was inevitably influenced by several factors:

- The number, consistency, and quality of reports (weight of publications)

Table 2
Diagnostic criteria for histologic phenotypes

Diagnosis	QL/QT	Minimum[a]	Adjunctive	Findings (brief)
Neuropathies				
1.1.1 Aganglionosis	QL, QT	H&E or EH	EH (AChE)	Complete absence of neurons
		IHC (calretinin)[b]		Hypertrophic submucosal extrinsic nerves
1.2.1 Hypoganglionosis	QL	H&E	IHC (PGP9.5, NSE)[b]	Severe reduction in ganglia and neurons
1.3.1 Ganglioneuromatosis	QL	H&E	IHC (PGP9.5, NSE, S100)[b]	Hamartomatous increase in neurons and glia
1.3.2 IND, type B	QT	EH (LDH)		More than eight neurons in >20% of 25 submucosal ganglia
1.4 Degenerative neuropathy	QL	H&E		Degenerative cytologic appearances
1.5 Inflammatory neuropathies	QL	H&E		Gross infiltrates or eosinophils
	QT	IHC (CD45, CD3)		One or more intraganglionic or more than five periganglionic lymphocytes/ganglion
1.6 Abnormal content	QL	H&E	IHC (SUMO1), TEM	Intraneuronal nuclear inclusion bodies in neurons
				Megamitochondria
		—	IHC (alpha-synuclein)[g]	Lewy bodies
1.7 Abnormal neurochemical coding	QL, QT	IHC[c]		Decreased immunostaining vs controls
		IHC[c]	IHC (PGP9.5, NSE)[bd]	Reduced defined subset of neurons
1.8 Neuronal immaturity	QL	H&E	EH (LDH, SDH)	Morphologically immature neurons
1.9 Abnormal enteric glia	QL	H&E	IHC (S100, GFAP)	Marked increase
Myopathies				
2.1 Muscularis propria	QL, QT	H&E	IHC (SMA, FLNA[g])	Any departure from two muscle layers malformations
2.2.1 Degen. leiomyopathy	QL	H&E	Tinctorial,[e] IHC (SMA) TEM	Myocyte damage and loss, fibrosis

(*continued on next page*)

Table 2
(continued)

Diagnosis	QL/QT	Minimum[a]	Adjunctive	Findings (brief)
2.2.2 Inflam. leiomyopathy	QL	H&E		Inflammatory cell infiltrate
2.3.1 *M. mucosae* hyperplasia	QL	H&E		Increased thickness musc. mucosae
2.4.1 Filament protein abnormalities	QL	IHC (SMA)		Absent SMA in circular muscle[f]
2.4.2 Inclusion bodies	QL, QT	H&E		Amphophilic "M" bodies
		Tinctorial (PAS)		Polyglucosan bodies
		TEM	IHC (antimitochondrial)[g]	Megamitochondria in myocytes
2.5.1 Atrophic desmosis	QL	Tinctorial[e]		Total or focal lack of connective tissue scaffold
Mesenchymopathies				
3.1 Abnormal ICC networks	QT	IHC (CD117)	IHC (Ano-1)	>50% reduced ICC in comparison with control sections

Abbreviations: AChE, acetylcholinesterase; Ano1 syn, DOG1; CD117 syn, c-kit; EH, enzyme histochemistry; FLNA, filamin A; H&E, hematoxylin and eosin; ICC, interstitial cells of Cajal; IHC, immunohistochemistry; IND, intestinal neuronal dysplasia; LDH, lactate dehydrogenase; PAS, periodic acid Schiff; QL, qualitative; QT, quantitative; SDH, succinate dehydrogenase; SMA, smooth muscle alpha actin; TEM, transmission electron microscopy.

[a] As recommended by IWG guidelines,[2] well oriented sections are required at a minimum of three levels through an appropriately fixed and oriented block.

[b] General neural markers used for comparison (Hu C/D, Neurofilament are alternatives).

[c] Undefined by IWG; most commonly employed are NO, ChAT, SP, VIP. Note: although provisionally included, these were not a recommendation of the IWG guidelines for general pathology practice.

[d] Panneuronal markers are used in this context to determine whether absolute numbers of neurons are reduced.

[e] Trichrome, Van Gieson, or picrosirius stain.

[f] Region specificity: this is a normal finding in ileum.

[g] Addition since 2010 publication (see text).

Modified from Knowles CH, De Giorgio R, Kapur RP, et al. The London Classification of gastrointestinal neuromuscular pathology: report on behalf of the Gastro 2009 International Working Group. Gut 2010;59(7):882–7; with permission.

- Sensitivity of the finding within these reports, that is, what proportion of patients with a clinical entity had the histologic feature
- Specificity of the finding to a single clinical entity (rather than to many clinical syndromes)
- Supportive basic science, particularly comparative animal models.

There were thus some areas where consensus was "rough" rather than unanimous. For this and other reasons, the London Classification was necessarily viewed as a starting point for future modification as new data became available. This review highlights some ongoing relational challenges and also some modifications that have already become necessary since 2010.

IMPACT ON PATIENT MANAGEMENT OR PROGNOSIS

Aside from the diagnosis of HSCR, there are few other well documented instances in which biopsy diagnoses definitely alter clinical care. Thus the number of patients for which specific therapy can be guided by histopathology is currently limited, for example, using immunosuppressants in diseases characterized by an underlying inflammatory phenotype.[10,11] Nevertheless, a histopathologic diagnosis can provide valuable insight into the etiology or pathogenesis of some forms of GI neuromuscular disorder (GINMD), which may afford important prognostic value, affect genetic counseling, and direct[12] and prevent[13] additional procedures. One of the other important functions of histopathologic studies in clinical management is the exclusion of particular phenotypes such as overt myopathy or associated phenotypes such as amyloidosis. The IWG defined reporting recommendations to provide for instances in which a "critical" diagnosis might acutely affect management.[2]

CLINICAL SCOPE

A complete review of all clinical entities associated with GI neuromuscular pathology is not possible in this article. Diseases in which dysmotility is not the central clinical characteristic (eg, Crohn's disease; radiation enteropathy; and tumors of nerve, smooth muscle, and ICC) have thus been excluded. Further, other local or systemic conditions with sequelae that include neuromuscular dysfunction, but in which the diagnostic utility of histopathology is questionable, have also been excluded, for example, acute conditions such as postoperative ileus and acute colonic pseudo-obstruction; disease entities with established macroscopic findings, for example, infantile hypertrophic pyloric stenosis, atresias, anorectal malformations, and megacystis–microcolon–hypoperistalsis syndrome; and other systemic diseases leading to sensorimotor dysfunction such as idiopathic autonomic neuropathy, Chagas' disease, human immunodeficiency virus (HIV), and amyloid-associated neuropathy in which intestinal full-thickness biopsies are rarely undertaken if the primary cause is known. Finally, because it has a specific and sizeable literature elsewhere, HSCR (although undoubtedly one of the more common and important enteric neuromuscular disorders) has also been excluded from this review. Digestive motility disorders have been defined throughout on a physiologic measurement basis in accord with the Bangkok classification[14] with a focus almost exclusively on "well defined entities." Both primary and secondary motility disturbances are addressed.

RESULTS BY CLINICAL ENTITY AND SITE

The main findings are presented by GI region, acknowledging that some disorders have a more general distribution. Where possible, the discussion has focused on data that have become available since publication of the first iteration of the London Classification and on challenges that persist in the field.

Primary Disorders

Esophagus

Summary

- Relevant clinical entities: idiopathic achalasia
- Tissue available: myectomy specimens from lower esophageal sphincter (LES)
- Histopathologic phenotypes from London Classification
  - Etiologic: hypoganglionosis or aganglionosis ± degenerative neuropathy ± lymphocytic or eosinophilic ganglionitis ± abnormal neurochemical coding (nitric oxide synthase [nNOS])
  - Morphologic: reduced ICC networks.

Discussion Full-thickness tissue is now less commonly available because of modern endoscopic therapies and is rarely a diagnostic requirement (based on manometric, radiologic, and endoscopic findings) (see article by Roman and Kahrilas elsewhere in this issue for further exploration of this topic). Histologic findings in achalasia are limited almost exclusively to neuropathies[15,16] where hypoganglionosis or aganglionosis of the LES, with or without degenerative or inflammatory features, are considered "etiologic." There is also reasonable evidence that specific neurochemically defined (functional) subsets of myenteric intrinsic motor neurons are preferentially lost, especially those coded for neuronal nNOS.[17,18] The finding of dense inflammatory infiltrates[19] in an adult with recent symptom onset should prompt a search for occult malignancy leading to paraneoplastic auto-antibody formation (see later).

Stomach

Summary

- Relevant clinical entities: idiopathic gastroparesis
- Tissue available: full-thickness corpus biopsies; rarely, partial gastrectomy
- Histopathologic phenotypes from London Classification (morphologic only): abnormal neurochemical coding (nNOS); abnormal ICC networks.

Discussion At the time of IWG consensus, the few data on gastroparesis were mostly limited to secondary disorders and case reports.[20,21] The recent vogue for gastric electrical stimulation (Enterra, Medtronic, Minneapolis, MN, USA) has provided an opportunity for the National Institutes of Health Gastroparesis Clinical Research Consortium to study 20 full-thickness biopsies taken at the time of lead implantation.[22] Cellular changes were compared with 20 controls from patients undergoing bariatric procedures (and 20 with diabetic gastroparesis; see later) using some standard histological and some research oriented techniques. Only 3/20 patients had evidence of neuropathy with neuronal drop out and decreased nerve fibers; however, 8/20 had selective nNOS neuronal loss. The most common histologic abnormality was a decrease in ICC, as identified by Kit immunolabeling, with 10 patients having a greater than 25% decrease in Kit expression. Both findings were consistent with previous reports and IWG consensus. The second most common abnormality noted was altered immune cells in the muscularis propria. This previously unreported finding was determined by immunolabeling against CD45; immune cells were abnormal in 8 patients on visual grading, all of whom had an infiltrate in the myenteric plexus region.

Small intestine

Summary

- Relevant clinical entities: chronic intestinal pseudo-obstruction (CIPO); enteric dysmotility
- Tissue available: full-thickness small bowel biopsies (most data on laparoscopic proximal jejunal biopsies[4,5,23]), rarely resection specimens
- Histopathologic phenotypes from London Classification
  - Congenital CIPO
    - Etiologic: aganglionosis, hypoganglionosis ± intraneuronal nuclear inclusions, degenerative neuropathy, muscularis propria malformations, and degenerative leiomyopathy
    - Morphologic: abnormal neurochemical coding, neuronal immaturity, and abnormal ICC networks
  - Acquired CIPO and enteric dysmotility
    - Etiologic: hypoganglionosis ± degenerative neuropathy ± lymphocytic or eosinophilic ganglionitis ± abnormal neurochemical coding, degenerative leiomyopathy ± lymphocytic or eosinophilic leiomyositis
    - Morphologic: increased glia, abnormal ICC networks, filament protein abnormalities, and polyglucosan inclusion bodies.

Discussion There is a clinical dichotomy among patients with CIPO that is reflected, to some extent, by histologic findings. Those patients with significant and persistent visceral dilatation from birth or infancy have a severe phenotype that may affect other hollow viscera and have a poor prognosis (50% mortality in childhood).[24] This group typically have well defined myopathies[25–27] and some neuropathies[13,28,29] that are readily diagnosed (with experience) on routine staining, may be familial,[25] and that may, in some cases, have a defined genetic etiology.[30,31] Such information is important for prognostic discussions and, sometimes, genetic counseling. One important clarification concerns the histologic features of X-linked CIPO, a rare disorder caused by mutations in the gene encoding the cytoskeletal protein filamin A (FLNA). This was previously considered to be a hereditary neuropathy on the basis of incomplete data.[32] Recent systematic study of two large families using contemporary methods now suggests that the mutation instead leads to abnormal lamination of the muscularis propria (**Fig. 1**) and thus a mainly myopathic basis for symptoms.[27]

Such patients contrast with those whose symptoms start in adulthood. These patients typically have severe chronic pain concomitant with symptoms suggesting retardation of intestinal transit, for example, nausea, vomiting, abdominal distension, and constipation. Evidence of transient or persistent radiologic visceral dilatation may or may not be present, providing the, perhaps theoretical, distinction between CIPO and enteric dysmotility, the latter having abnormal small bowel manometry only.[33,34] Both disorders are challenging histologically because most easily defined phenotypes in congenital CIPO, with fibrosis and vacuolation, are infrequent, for example, gross myopathies.[4,5] Whether CIPO and enteric dysmotility represent discrete entities continues to be debated, with some evidence to support such a division from recent histopathologic observations made on a series of 115 full-thickness jejunal biopsies.[5] In this study, patients with CIPO were more likely to have myopathies (22% vs 5%)

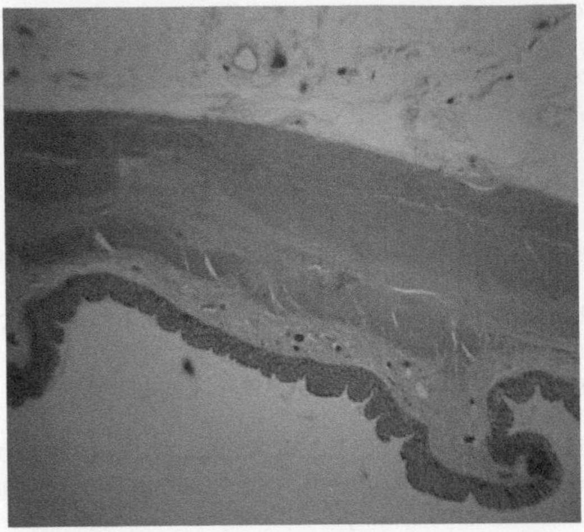

Fig. 1. Reduplication of circular layer of the muscularis propria in a patient with intestinal pseudo-obstruction (hematoxylin and eosin staining).

and less likely to have inflammatory neuropathy (26% vs 69%; **Fig. 2**). From a biological mechanism perspective, the reporting of inflammation with neuronal degeneration and increased enteric glia[35] in patients whose predominant symptom is unexplained chronic pain may also have clinical relevance because these findings constitute the neuropathic pain triad.[36] Morphine is an activator of microglia and long-standing, high-dose opioid use may have led to visceral hyperalgesia in some patients.[37]

Colon

Summary

- Relevant clinical entities: slow-transit constipation (STC) and idiopathic megacolon/megarectum

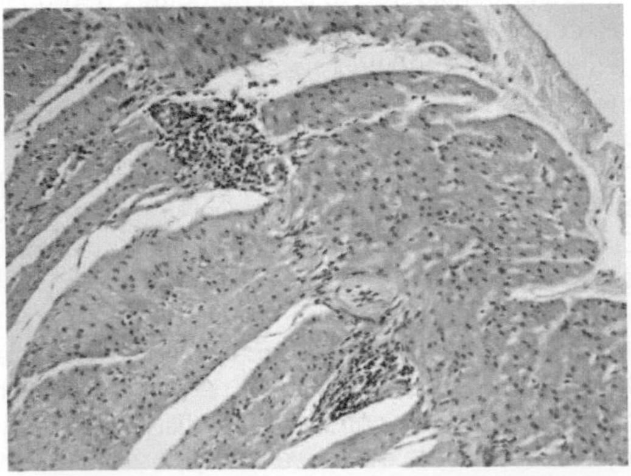

Fig. 2. Focal lymphocytic plexitis of the myenteric plexus in a patient with enteric dysmotility (hematoxylin and eosin staining).

- Tissue available: colonic resection specimens, laparoscopic seromuscular biopsies,[38,39] some data also on laparoscopic proximal jejunal biopsies[40]
- Histopathologic phenotypes from London Classification
  - Slow transit constipation (all morphologic) hypoganglionosis ± degenerative neuropathy ± abnormal neurochemical coding, intestinal neuronal dysplasia type B (IND-type B), lymphocytic ganglionitis, abnormal ICC networks, amphophilic inclusion bodies
  - Idiopathic megacolon (all morphologic) hypoganglionosis ± degenerative neuropathy, IND-type B, abnormal neurochemical coding, degenerative leiomyopathy, muscularis mucosae hypertrophy, filament protein abnormalities, atrophic desmosis.

Discussion The diagnosis of colonic histologic abnormalities in patients with STC has been very recently reviewed in detail[41] and has considerable overlap with idiopathic megacolon. The two ongoing main challenges concern the diagnosis of neuropathy (in terms of whether it is present or not) and that of reduced ICC networks (in terms of the significance of the finding).

A diagnosis of neuropathy is fraught with methodological and interpretive issues including patient selection, type of surgery (and influence that this may have had on findings), staining methods (especially data from outdated neuronal methods, e.g., silver staining), and lack of normative data. On this basis it can be concluded that reductions in absolute number or degeneration of enteric neurons, despite extensive reporting thereof,[42–44] are probably not common findings based on current diagnostic criteria.[41] Abnormal neurochemical coding has also been studied extensively; however, few studies have concurrently used a pan-neuronal marker to determine whether observed changes represent an absolute reduction in number of a particular neurochemically defined subset of neurons. The most robust of these findings details significant reductions in cholinergic and increases in nitrergic neuron subpopulations,[45] findings that corroborate in vitro studies[46,47] and responses to novel drugs.[48]

Even more contentious is the diagnosis of IND-type B. IND-type B is a highly controversial entity in children and, where diagnosed, has been presumed to account for symptoms such as chronic constipation with or without colonic dilatation.[49,50] ENS changes include an increased density of submucosal ganglia, based on the finding of more than 8 neurons in 20% or more of at least 25 ganglia, and have been established only with lactate dehydrogenase enzyme histochemistry in 15-μm-thick frozen sections. No analogous quantitative criteria exist for the recognition of "giant" submucosal ganglia in H&E or immunohistochemically stained paraffin sections and the influence of age and site of biopsy on normative data contribute to significant problems of diagnostic certainty.

There is an abundance of data (11 studies) published in the last decade demonstrating reductions in ICC in patients with STC.[41,51–53] In contrast to neuropathy, nearly all studies have been performed on well characterized patients with physiologically defined STC, and although there are some methodological issues in terms of immunohistochemical methods of antigen retrieval and visualization,[54] there is little doubt that reduced ICC is the most consistent histologic finding in STC to date. The widespread association of decreased ICC in several other digestive motility disorders (see earlier) raises the issue of whether ICC loss is part of the primary disease (etiologic) or is secondary to a subsequent insult such as inflammation or obstruction (morphologic). Inflammation[55] and obstruction[56] have both been shown in animal models to be associated with reversible loss of Kit-positive ICC. Whether this reflects actual death of the cell remains unclear and is, probably, unlikely. ICCs are also susceptible to ischemia and care must be taken to minimize ischemia when collecting human specimens.[57] This is particularly relevant with laparoscopic surgery in which the blood supply is often cut off a substantial time before the tissue is extracted.

Secondary Disorders

A variety of systemic diseases can lead to disordered GI motility. A role for histologic study of GI tissues as a guide to diagnosis or treatment is currently very limited and probably applies only to rare mitochondrial disorders, paraneoplastic syndromes, and Parkinson's disease–related dysmotility. Diabetes and scleroderma have been included, although it is acknowledged that these represent areas where pathology is more likely only to guide developments of new therapies based on understanding of disease biology rather than influence current management of the individual patient.

Mitochondrial encephalomyopathies

Summary

- Relevant clinical entities: intestinal pseudo-obstruction, chronic constipation, megacolon, visceral perforation
- Tissue available: small bowel and rectal biopsies (resection/autopsy specimens)
  - Histopathologic phenotypes from London Classification (etiologic only): megamitochondria.

Mitochondrial encephalomyopathies are a heterogeneous group of genetic disorders caused by dysfunction of the mitochondrial respiratory chain.[58] Among mitochondrial encephalomyopathies, the one most frequently associated with GI dysmotility and CIPO is mitochondrial neurogastrointestinal encephalomyopathy (MNGIE), an autosomal recessive syndrome due to mutations in the thymidine phosphorylase gene *TYMP*[59] resulting in depletion of mitochondrial DNA[60] and compensatory mitochondrial proliferation. The latter are evident histologically as inclusion bodies (megamitochondria), especially in the longitudinal smooth muscle, with accompanying degeneration and thinning of the muscularis propria. Although diagnosis is largely dependent on clinical suspicion, magnetic resonance imaging (MRI) of the brain, and enzyme assays in blood and skeletal muscle, several cases have been reported in which histology has contributed to the diagnosis.[61,62]

Paraneoplastic gastroenteropathy

Summary

- Relevant clinical entities: (pseudo)achalasia, gastroparesis, intestinal pseudo-obstruction
- Tissue available: gastric and small bowel biopsies (occasionally resection specimens)
- Histopathologic phenotypes from London Classification
  - Etiologic: hypoganglionosis or aganglionosis ± lymphocytic ganglionitis and/or leiomyositis
  - Morphologic: increased glia.

Discussion Autoimmune GI motor dysfunction can be associated with small cell carcinoma of the lung (SCLC) and other neoplasms with or without coexisting neurologic disorders including peripheral neuropathies and autonomic dysfunction, cerebellar degeneration, and limbic encephalitis.[63–65] Histologic examination of GI tissue from patients with paraneoplastic motility disorders reveals myenteric ganglionitis/plexitis including lymphocytic and plasma cellular infiltration, enteroglial cell proliferation, neuronal degeneration, and loss and progression to aganglionosis in the most severe cases.[63,66,67] GI symptoms often precede diagnosis of tumor.[64,66] Thus GI symptoms ± histology may provoke the search for several potentially pathogenic paraneoplastic autoantibodies that, if identified, strongly suggest the presence of an underlying malignancy. Of these, type 1 antineuronal nuclear antibodies (ANNA-1), also referred to as anti-Hu (based on the molecular target), recognize a family of RNA binding proteins expressed by central and peripheral neurones, including enteric neurones and SCLC tumor cells.[68]ANNA-1 are found in the majority of patients with paraneoplastic neurologic syndromes secondary to SCLC[64,69] and, similarly, provide a useful serologic marker for SCLC-related paraneoplastic GI dysmotility.[66] Other antibodies targeting cell-surface channels/receptors have been detected in smaller numbers of cases of paraneoplastic GI dysmotility, including anti-N-type voltage gated calcium channels (VGCCs) associated with SCLC, retroperitoneal B-cell lymphoma and ovarian carcinoma,[66] P/Q-type VGCCs (as in Lambert Eaton myasthenic syndrome) with SCLC and ganglionic $\alpha 3$ nicotinic acetylcholine receptors (as in idiopathic and paraneoplastic autonomic neuropathies) with SCLC, thymoma, and bladder and rectal carcinoma.[70] Specific immunologic therapies may be thus directed.[10,11]

Parkinson's disease
Summary

- Relevant clinical entities: mainly chronic constipation
- Tissue available: deep submucosal endoscopic biopsies (postmortem tissues)
  - Histopathologic phenotypes from London Classification: none (not included).

Discussion Parkinson's disease was not included within the London Classification but is worthy of mention because recent data suggest that histopathology of the ENS may provide a "window" to similar changes in the CNS and thus have some role as a biomarker for disease.[71,72] This would be impractical were it not for the fact that the main pathognomonic finding, that of Lewy bodies and neuritis, may be detectable in deep submucosal biopsies attained at colonoscopy.[73,74] In a recent study, Lewy pathology was diagnosed in 21/29 Parkinson's disease patients but in none of 10 controls.[73] Although this required use of a nonstandard antibody (alpha-synuclein) as well as standard (IWG recommended) immunostains to count neurons, for example, neurofilament, the authors rightly concluded that the technique may by a useful tool for premortem neuropathologic diagnosis of Parkinson's disease and monitoring of progression.

Diabetic gastroenteropathy
Summary

- Relevant clinical entities: gastroparesis, chronic constipation
- Tissue available: gastric corpus biopsies and a lesser number of gastrectomy specimens, colonic resections[75]
- Histopathologic phenotypes from London Classification
  - Etiologic: abnormal neurochemical coding (deficiency of nNOS-containing neurons), abnormal ICC networks
  - Morphologic: degenerative neuropathy, amphophilic inclusion bodies.

Discussion Diabetes mellitus is well recognized to lead to neuronal injury. Effects on the GI tract are presumably diffuse although clinical entities most commonly implicate the stomach, colon, and anorectum. The contribution of extrinsic (autonomic) versus intrinsic (ENS) neuronal dysfunction to clinical syndromes is difficult to quantify. There is, however, support for the latter in relation to the stomach, in which recent controlled data from the Gastroparesis Clinical Research Consortium has confirmed the IWG view and previous reports[76] that neuropathy characterized by loss of nNOS coded neurons (4/20 patients) and reduced ICC networks (10/20 patients) can be considered etiologic. In common with idiopathic gastroparesis, a proportion of patients (8/20) also had immune cell infiltrate in the myenteric plexus region.[22] It is noted that these findings are corroborated by extensive studies in diabetic rodent models.[77]

Connective tissue gastroenteropathy

Summary

- Relevant clinical entities: achalasia, megacolon
- Tissue available: rare biopsy and resection specimens (postmortem tissues)
  - Histopathologic phenotypes from London Classification (etiologic only) degenerative leiomyopathy.

Severe bowel dysfunction occurs in a proportion of patients with connective tissue disorders and is most commonly associated with systemic sclerosis (scleroderma). GI symptoms may be the presenting symptoms for the diagnosis and may precede the actual diagnosis by months to years. Any region of the gut may be affected, although esophageal dysmotility is most commonly recognized.[78] The pathophysiologic mechanism appears to be one of smooth muscle atrophy and, to a lesser degree, fibrosis,[79,80] with an immunologic component suggested by the observation of a range of disease-specific antibodies.[81–83] Diagnosis and treatment are, however, rarely, if ever, influenced by knowledge by histologic findings.

SUMMARY

The recent development of consensus guidelines for the preparation and staining of tissues, the publication of the London Classification, and reviews of what is normal in the enteric neuromusculature have been significant steps forward in this field.[1–3] Increased accessibility to full-thickness biopsies of the bowel wall facilitated by advances in laparoscopic surgery have also played a part in making the decision to ask for a tissue diagnosis easier. Better antibodies for immunohistochemistry and a better understanding of disease processes at work, such as those seen in filamin mutations, all help inform the range of information that can be gleaned from what is usually a very limited sample. Clinical phenotyping remains difficult in many patients, but the availability of specialist pathologic review and the standardization of staining between laboratories are leading to better defined histologic phenotypes, that inform, in turn, possible biological processes at work in these patients. In many instances, a diagnosis may come to light only after some time, and the retention of pathologic samples in paraffin wax, as is standard practice in most laboratories, is of great value in reassessing samples, often after many years, in the light of new advances. The highest quality information, and the best answer for the patient, is, as ever, achieved by close working relationships and excellent communication between clinicians and pathologists.

REFERENCES

1. Knowles CH, De Giorgio R, Kapur RP, et al. The London Classification of gastrointestinal neuromuscular pathology: report on behalf of the Gastro 2009 International Working Group. Gut 2010;59(7):882–7.

2. Knowles CH, De Giorgio R, Kapur RP, et al. Gastrointestinal neuromuscular pathology: guidelines for histological techniques and reporting on behalf of the Gastro 2009 International Working Group. Acta Neuropathol 2009;118(2):271–301.
3. Knowles CH, Veress B, Kapur RP, et al. Quantitation of cellular components of the enteric nervous system in the normal human gastrointestinal tract—report on behalf of the Gastro 2009 International Working Group. Neurogastroenterol Motil 2011;23(2):115–24.
4. Knowles CH, Veress B, Tornblom H, et al. Safety and diagnostic yield of laparoscopically assisted full-thickness bowel biospy. Neurogastroenterol Motil 2008;20(7):774–9.
5. Lindberg G, Tornblom H, Iwarzon M, et al. Full-thickness biopsy findings in chronic intestinal pseudo-obstruction and enteric dysmotility. Gut 2009;58(8):1084–90.
6. Fitzgibbons PL, Chandrasoma PT. Familial visceral myopathy. Evidence of diffuse involvement of intestinal smooth muscle. Am J Surg Pathol 1987;11(11):846–54.
7. Martin JE, Hester TW, Aslam H, et al. Discordant practice and limited histopathological assessment in gastrointestinal neuromuscular disease. Gut 2009;58(12):1703–5.
8. Swaminathan M, Kapur RP. Counting myenteric ganglion cells in histologic sections: an empirical approach. Hum Pathol 2010;41(8):1097–1108.
9. Scott SM, Knowles CH, Wang D, et al. The nocturnal jejunal migrating motor complex: defining normal ranges by study of 51 healthy adult volunteers and meta-analysis. Neurogastroenterol Motil 2006;18(10):927–35.
10. De Giorgio R, Barbara G, Stanghellini V, et al. Clinical and morphofunctional features of idiopathic myenteric ganglionitis underlying severe intestinal motor dysfunction: a study of three cases. Am J Gastroenterol 2002;97(9):2454–9.
11. Pasha SF, Lunsford TN, Lennon VA. Autoimmune gastrointestinal dysmotility treated successfully with pyridostigmine. Gastroenterology 2006;131(5):1592–6.
12. Hubball A, Martin JE, Lang B, et al. The role of humoral autoimmunity in gastrointestinal neuromuscular diseases. Prog Neurobiol 2009;87(1):10–20.
13. Heneyke S, Smith VV, Spitz L, et al. Chronic intestinal pseudo-obstruction: treatment and long term follow up of 44 patients. Arch Dis Child 1999;81(1):21–7.
14. Wingate DL. "Functional" should not be shorthand for "I don't know" in dyspepsia. BMJ 2002;324(7333):364.
15. Csendes A, Smok G, Braghetto I, et al. Histological studies of Auerbach's plexuses of the oesophagus, stomach, jejunum, and colon in patients with achalasia of the oesophagus: correlation with gastric acid secretion, presence of parietal cells and gastric emptying of solids. Gut 1992;33(2):150–4.
16. Goldblum JR, Rice TW, Richter JE. Histopathologic features in esophagomyotomy specimens from patients with achalasia. Gastroenterology 1996;111(3):648–54.
17. Zarate N, Wang XY, Tougas G, et al. Intramuscular interstitial cells of Cajal associated with mast cells survive nitrergic nerves in achalasia. Neurogastroenterol Motil 2006;18(7):556–68.
18. Gockel I, Bohl JR, Eckardt VF, et al. Reduction of interstitial cells of Cajal (ICC) associated with neuronal nitric oxide synthase (n-NOS) in patients with achalasia. Am J Gastroenterol 2008;103(4):856–64.
19. Clark SB, Rice TW, Tubbs RR, et al. The nature of the myenteric infiltrate in achalasia: an immunohistochemical analysis. Am J Surg Pathol 2000;24(8):1153–8.
20. Ejskjaer NT, Bradley JL, Buxton-Thomas MS, et al. Novel surgical treatment and gastric pathology in diabetic gastroparesis. Diabet Med 1999;16(6):488–95.
21. Zarate N, Mearin F, Wang XY, et al. Severe idiopathic gastroparesis due to neuronal and interstitial cells of Cajal degeneration: pathological findings and management. Gut 2003;52(7):966–70.

22. Grover M, Farrugia G, Lurken MS, et al. Cellular changes in diabetic and idiopathic gastroparesis. Gastroenterology 2011;140(5):1575–85, e1578.
23. Knowles CH, Silk DB, Darzi A, et al. Deranged smooth muscle alpha-actin as a biomarker of intestinal pseudo-obstruction: a controlled multinational case series. Gut 2004;53(11):1583–9.
24. Rudolph CD, Hyman PE, Altschuler SM, et al. Diagnosis and treatment of chronic intestinal pseudo-obstruction in children: report of consensus workshop. J Pediatr Gastroenterol Nutr 1997;24(1):102–12.
25. Schuffler MD, Lowe MC, Bill AH. Studies of idiopathic intestinal pseudoobstruction. I. Hereditary hollow visceral myopathy: clinical and pathological studies. Gastroenterology 1977;73(2):327–38.
26. Smith VV, Milla PJ. Histological phenotypes of enteric smooth muscle disease causing functional intestinal obstruction in childhood. Histopathology 1997;31(2): 112–22.
27. Kapur RP, Robertson SP, Hannibal MC, et al. Diffuse abnormal layering of small intestinal smooth muscle is present in patients with FLNA mutations and X-linked intestinal pseudo-obstruction. Am J Surg Pathol 2010;34(10):1528–43.
28. Rudin C, Jenny P, Ohnacker H, et al. Absence of the enteric nervous system in the newborn: presentation of three patients and review of the literature. J Pediatr Surg 1986;21(4):313–8.
29. Navarro J, Sonsino E, Boige N, et al. Visceral neuropathies responsible for chronic intestinal pseudo-obstruction syndrome in pediatric practice: analysis of 26 cases. J Pediatr Gastroenterol Nutr 1990;11(2):179–95.
30. Pingault V, Girard M, Bondurand N, et al. SOX10 mutations in chronic intestinal pseudo-obstruction suggest a complex physiopathological mechanism. Hum Genet 2002;111(2):198–206.
31. Deglincerti A, De Giorgio R, Cefle K, et al. A novel locus for syndromic chronic idiopathic intestinal pseudo-obstruction maps to chromosome 8q23–q24. Eur J Hum Genet 2007;15(8):889–97.
32. Auricchio A, Brancolini V, Casari G, et al. The locus for a novel syndromic form of neuronal intestinal pseudoobstruction maps to Xq28. Am J Hum Genet 1996;58(4): 743–8.
33. Wingate D, Hongo M, Kellow J, et al. Disorders of gastrointestinal motility: towards a new classification. J Gastroenterol Hepatol 2002;17(Suppl):S1–14.
34. Lindberg G, Iwarzon M, Tornblom H. Clinical features and long-term survival in chronic intestinal pseudo-obstruction and enteric dysmotility. Scand J Gastroenterol 2009; 44(6):692–9.
35. Schuffler MD, Jonak Z. Chronic idiopathic intestinal pseudo-obstruction caused by a degenerative disorder of the myenteric plexus: the use of Smith's method to define the neuropathology. Gastroenterology 1982;82(3):476–86.
36. Scholz J, Woolf CJ. The neuropathic pain triad: neurons, immune cells and glia. Nat Neurosci 2007;10(11):1361–8.
37. Olesen AE, Staahl C, Arendt-Nielsen L, et al. Different effects of morphine and oxycodone in experimentally evoked hyperalgesia: a human translational study. Br J Clin Pharmacol 2010;70(2):189–200.
38. King SK, Sutcliffe JR, Hutson JM. Laparoscopic seromuscular colonic biopsies: a surgeon's experience. J Pediatr Surg 2005;40(2):381–4.
39. Hutson JM, Chow CW, Borg J. Intractable constipation with a decrease in substance P-immunoreactive fibres: is it a variant of intestinal neuronal dysplasia? J Pediatr Surg 1996;31(4):580–3.

40. Veress B, Nyberg B, Tornblom H, et al. Intestinal lymphocytic epithelioganglionitis: a unique combination of inflammation in bowel dysmotility: a histopathological and immunohistochemical analysis of 28 cases. Histopathology 2009;54(5):539–49.
41. Knowles CH, Farrugia G. Gastrointestinal neuromuscular pathology in chronic constipation. Best Pract Res Clin Gastroenterol 2011;25(1):43–57.
42. Smith B, Grace RH, Todd IP. Organic constipation in adults. Br J Surg 1977;64(5): 313–4.
43. Krishnamurthy S, Schuffler MD, Rohrmann CA, et al. Severe idiopathic constipation is associated with a distinctive abnormality of the colonic myenteric plexus. Gastroenterology 1985;88(1 Pt 1):26–34.
44. Porter AJ, Wattchow DA, Hunter A, et al. Abnormalities of nerve fibers in the circular muscle of patients with slow transit constipation. Int J Colorectal Dis 1998;13(5–6): 208–16.
45. Wattchow D, Brookes S, Murphy E, et al. Regional variation in the neurochemical coding of the myenteric plexus of the human colon and changes in patients with slow transit constipation. Neurogastroenterol Motil 2008;20(12):1298–1305.
46. Burleigh DE. Evidence for a functional cholinergic deficit in human colonic tissue resected for constipation. J Pharm Pharmacol 1988;40(1):55–7.
47. Mitolo-Chieppa D, Mansi G, Rinaldi R, et al. Cholinergic stimulation and nonadrenergic, noncholinergic relaxation of human colonic circular muscle in idiopathic chronic constipation. Dig Dis Sci 1998;43(12):2719–26.
48. Camilleri M, Kerstens R, Rykx A, et al. A placebo-controlled trial of prucalopride for severe chronic constipation. N Engl J Med 2008;358(22):2344–54.
49. Scharli AF, Meier-Ruge W. Localized and disseminated forms of neuronal intestinal dysplasia mimicking Hirschsprung's disease. J Pediatr Surg 1981;16(2):164–70.
50. Koletzko S, Jesch I, Faus-Kebetaler T, et al. Rectal biopsy for diagnosis of intestinal neuronal dysplasia in children: a prospective multicentre study on interobserver variation and clinical outcome. Gut 1999;44(6):853–61.
51. He CL, Burgart L, Wang L, et al. Decreased interstitial cell of cajal volume in patients with slow-transit constipation. Gastroenterology 2000;118(1):14–21.
52. Lyford GL, He CL, Soffer E, et al. Pan-colonic decrease in interstitial cells of Cajal in patients with slow transit constipation. Gut 2002;51(4):496–501.
53. Wedel T, Spiegler J, Soellner S, et al. Enteric nerves and interstitial cells of Cajal are altered in patients with slow-transit constipation and megacolon. Gastroenterology 2002;123(5):1459–67.
54. Garrity MM, Gibbons SJ, Smyrk TC, et al. Diagnostic challenges of motility disorders: optimal detection of CD117+ interstitial cells of Cajal. Histopathology 2009;54(3): 286–94.
55. Der T, Bercik P, Donnelly G, et al. Interstitial cells of cajal and inflammation-induced motor dysfunction in the mouse small intestine. Gastroenterology 2000;119(6): 1590–9.
56. Chang IY, Glasgow NJ, Takayama I, et al. Loss of interstitial cells of Cajal and development of electrical dysfunction in murine small bowel obstruction. J Physiol (Lond) 2001;536(2):555–68.
57. Farrugia G. Interstitial cells of Cajal in health and disease. Neurogastroent Motil 2008;20:54–63.
58. DiMauro S, Schon EA. Mitochondrial respiratory-chain diseases. N Engl J Med 2003;348(26):2656–68.
59. Nishino I, Spinazzola A, Papadimitriou A, et al. Mitochondrial neurogastrointestinal encephalomyopathy: an autosomal recessive disorder due to thymidine phosphorylase mutations. Ann Neurol 2000;47(6):792–800.

60. Giordano C, Sebastiani M, De Giorgio R, et al. Gastrointestinal dysmotility in mitochondrial neurogastrointestinal encephalomyopathy is caused by mitochondrial DNA depletion. Am J Pathol 2008;173(4):1120–8.
61. Perez-Atayde AR, Fox V, Teitelbaum JE, et al. Mitochondrial neurogastrointestinal encephalomyopathy: diagnosis by rectal biopsy. Am J Surg Pathol 1998;22(9): 1141–7.
62. Muehlenberg K, Fiedler A, Schaumann I, et al. [Intestinal pseudoobstructions and gastric necrosis in mitochondrial myopathy]. Dtsch Med Wochenschr 2002;127(12): 611–5.
63. Chinn JS, Schuffler MD. Paraneoplastic visceral neuropathy as a cause of severe gastrointestinal motor dysfunction. Gastroenterology 1988;95(5):1279–86.
64. Lucchinetti CF, Kimmel DW, Lennon VA. Paraneoplastic and oncologic profiles of patients seropositive for type 1 antineuronal nuclear autoantibodies. Neurology 1998; 50(3):652–7.
65. Vernino S, Adamski J, Kryzer TJ, et al. Neuronal nicotinic ACh receptor antibody in subacute autonomic neuropathy and cancer-related syndromes. Neurology 1998; 50(6):1806–13.
66. Lee HR, Lennon VA, Camilleri M, et al. Paraneoplastic gastrointestinal motor dysfunction: clinical and laboratory characteristics. Am J Gastroenterol 2001;96(2):373–9.
67. Schuffler MD, Baird HW, Fleming CR, et al. Intestinal pseudo-obstruction as the presenting manifestation of small-cell carcinoma of the lung. A paraneoplastic neuropathy of the gastrointestinal tract. Ann Intern Med 1983;98(2):129–34.
68. Altermatt HJ, Rodriguez M, Scheithauer BW, et al. Paraneoplastic anti-Purkinje and type I anti-neuronal nuclear autoantibodies bind selectively to central, peripheral, and autonomic nervous system cells. Lab Invest 1991;65(4):412–20.
69. Lennon VA, Sas DF, Busk MF, et al. Enteric neuronal autoantibodies in pseudoobstruction with small-cell lung carcinoma. Gastroenterology 1991;100(1):137–42.
70. Vernino S, Low PA, Fealey RD, et al. Autoantibodies to ganglionic acetylcholine receptors in autoimmune autonomic neuropathies. N Engl J Med 2000;343(12):847–55.
71. Qualman SJ, Haupt HM, Yang P, Hamilton SR. Esophageal Lewy bodies associated with ganglion cell loss in achalasia. Similarity to Parkinson's disease. Gastroenterology 1984;87(4):848–56.
72. Braak H, Braak E. Pathoanatomy of Parkinson's disease. J Neurol 2000;247(Suppl 2):II3–10.
73. Lebouvier T, Neunlist M, Bruley des Varannes S, et al. Colonic biopsies to assess the neuropathology of Parkinson's disease and its relationship with symptoms. PLoS One 2010;5(9):e12728.
74. Lebouvier T, Chaumette T, Damier P, et al. Pathological lesions in colonic biopsies during Parkinson's disease. Gut 2008;57(12):1741–3.
75. Nakahara M, Isozaki K, Hirota S, et al. Deficiency of KIT-positive cells in the colon of patients with diabetes mellitus. J Gastroenterol Hepatol 2002;17(6):666–70.
76. He CL, Soffer EE, Ferris CD, et al. Loss of interstitial cells of Cajal and inhibitory innervation in insulin-dependent diabetes. Gastroenterology 2001;121(2):427–34.
77. Wang XY, Huizinga JD, Diamond J, et al. Loss of intramuscular and submuscular interstitial cells of Cajal and associated enteric nerves is related to decreased gastric emptying in streptozotocin-induced diabetes. Neurogastroenterol Motil 2009;21(10): 1095-e92.
78. Rose S, Young MA, Reynolds JC. Gastrointestinal manifestations of scleroderma. Gastroenterol Clin North Am 1998;27(3):563–94.

79. Schuffler MD, Beegle RG. Progressive systemic sclerosis of the gastrointestinal tract and hereditary hollow visceral myopathy: two distinguishable disorders of intestinal smooth muscle. Gastroenterology 1979;77(4 Pt 1):664–71.
80. Roberts CG, Hummers LK, Ravich WJ, et al. A case-control study of the pathology of oesophageal disease in systemic sclerosis (scleroderma). Gut 2006;55(12):1697–1703.
81. Hietarinta M, Ilonen J, Lassila O, et al. Association of HLA antigens with anti-Scl-70-antibodies and clinical manifestations of systemic sclerosis (scleroderma). Br J Rheumatol 1994;33(4):323–6.
82. Gilchrist FC, Bunn C, Foley PJ, et al. Class II HLA associations with autoantibodies in scleroderma: a highly significant role for HLA-DP. Genes Immun 2001;2(2):76–81.
83. Goldblatt F, Gordon TP, Waterman SA. Antibody-mediated gastrointestinal dysmotility in scleroderma. Gastroenterology 2002;123(4):1144–50.

A 21st Century Look at the Spectrum of Gastrointestinal Motility Disorders. What is Dysmotility; What is Functional?

Hans Törnblom, MD, PhD, Greger Lindberg, MD, PhD*

KEYWORDS

- Digestive physiology • Esophageal manometry
- Gastrointestinal motility • Functional colonic diseases
- Functional gastrointestinal disorders • Esophageal disease
- Signs and symptoms

Gastrointestinal motility disorders affect the neuromuscular functions needed for movement of contents through the gastrointestinal tract. This definition excludes strictures and other mechanical causes for impaired passage from the concept of motility disorders. Functional gastrointestinal disorders (FGID), on the other hand, have traditionally been believed to arise from a gastrointestinal tract with an intact neuromuscular function. Most definitions of FGID include the absence of structural changes, but the depth of the search for such changes has varied. The latest version of the Rome Criteria for functional bowel disorders states that "research will likely confirm that functional gut disorders manifest such (structural or biochemical) findings".[1]

Our view is that motility disorders and functional disorders should be regarded as 2 different vectors for classifying patients, one physiologic that relies on measuring dysmotility and the other a symptom vector describing the subjective sensations of disordered function. In some instances, symptoms follow from a well-defined state of dysmotility, which, in turn, can have a well-defined underlying pathology. This is the case, for example, with achalasia. The events leading to degeneration of nitric oxide producing neurons and the resultant inability of the lower esophageal sphincter to relax on swallowing, thus leading to dysphagia, chest pain, and regurgitation, are multiple and varied. Still, we recognize achalasia as a typical motility disorder. In other instances, symptoms like diarrhea or abdominal

The authors have nothing to disclose.

Karolinska Institutet, Department of Medicine, Karolinska University Hospital, SE-141 86, Stockholm, Sweden
* Corresponding author.
E-mail address: greger.lindberg@ki.se

Gastroenterol Clin N Am 40 (2011) 715–723
doi:10.1016/j.gtc.2011.09.011

distension cannot be ascribed to a particular physiologic disturbance, and our current methods do not allow us to detect an underlying pathology. This does not necessarily mean that no such pathology exists; it may instead reflect the inability of our current methods to detect abnormalities.

SYMPTOM-BASED DIAGNOSIS—THE FUNCTIONAL MAINSTAY

The perception of ill health reported by the patient when consulting a physician is the basis for all diagnostic decision making except in certain emergency situations. The combined outcome of how the individual physician judges the medical history and the results of diagnostic tests and treatment trials affects the way a diagnosis is seen. Traditionally, what cannot be seen, measured, or assessed by a positive treatment response is regarded as less confirmative of a "real" disease compared with diagnoses that are obvious from 1, or preferably all 3, of these viewpoints. Even if empiric treatment is the mode of diagnosis, we tend to accept it as proof for somatic disease without too much hesitance, as long as there is a symptom improvement, as is the case with acid suppression for reflux symptoms.

A major problem regarding the 28 adult FGIDs as defined today[2] is that most of them do not, in any convincing way, meet our traditional view of clinical diagnoses. In the first instance, the labeling of FGIDs as disorders creates some confusion because this is a common term in psychiatry but not in somatic medicine. The routine practice to exclude organic disease before making a diagnosis of a FGID further emphasizes this; rule out "diseases" and the "disorders" are what remains.

During the last 2 decades, the Rome process has changed our ways of thinking about FGIDs quite a lot. The Rome process started out by using consensus of opinion but has developed into a more-or-less worldwide scientific joint venture for creating evidence-based and improved knowledge regarding FGIDs. One of the objectives of the Rome process was to create the means for a positive diagnosis of FGIDs; exclusion of organic disease should no longer be needed. The message from Rome is that clusters of symptoms with a minimum duration of six months and without alarm symptoms can safely be used for diagnosing a benign disorder with a reasonably well-defined prognosis.[2] The dissemination of this strategy, in particular to community providers of health care, may still have a long way to go.[3] Although the stability over time of a given FGID is poor, with FGIDs tending to change labels, eg, from irritable bowel syndrome (IBS) to functional dyspepsia or functional constipation,[4,5] new organic diseases do not appear to develop more often than in the general population.[6–8] The major diagnostic drift stays within the framework defined by FGID.[4] The diagnostic certainty conveyed by symptom criteria is an important step forward in everyday work and a trustworthy basis on which to start in the therapeutic relation with a patient.

Several problems seem inherent to FGID. To start with, those who seek medical advice for FGID have either more severe symptoms than nonconsulting FGID patients or carry more psychological problems, like anxiety, depression, somatization, and general health concerns.[9] It is vital to understand the patient's reasons for seeking medical advice and to also address contributing factors. Medical therapy for FGIDs is hampered by the lack of efficacious drugs. Symptomatic treatment for patients with diagnoses of unknown etiology and uncertain pathophysiology is a challenge. A confident and skilled physician seems to increase the chance for improvement, even if the treatment modes are not particularly effective.[7,10] This is exemplified by the high placebo response to treatment interventions in IBS,[11] which is good for short-term success but may increase the risk for continued use of ineffective drugs unless careful follow-up is performed.

PHYSIOLOGY-BASED DIAGNOSIS

The diagnosis of dysmotility requires some means for measuring motor activity of the gastrointestinal tract. Any such measurement, in turn, requires that the boundaries of normal motility are known, and that this measurement is performed using an agreed upon or standardized technique. This is where the concept of physiology-based diagnosis starts to become complicated. Measurement techniques are constantly evolving, and only a few techniques have finally made it into clinical practice. The market for measurement systems is relatively small, and, although producers of measurement instruments aim for solutions that will sell enough numbers of units to make a profit, they depend on medical researchers and research groups for defining clinically relevant measures. In many areas of gastrointestinal physiology, it has been difficult to establish clinical relevance. A typical example is electrogastrography, ie, the measurement of gastric electrical activity from cutaneous electrodes. Despite developments in hardware and software for automated signal analysis, the clinical relevance of measuring gastric electrical activity has remained unproven.[12] Expertise in a number of techniques, such as 3-dimensional ultrasonography for gastric accommodation and emptying[13] and intraluminal manometry of the left colon, has been confined to a few groups.[14,15] At any given point it has been very difficult to predict the winners among currently available techniques.

As a corollary, only a few measurement techniques have gained widespread use. These include 24-hour pH-monitoring of esophageal exposure to acidic reflux, esophageal manometry, gastric emptying using a radionuclide-labeled meal, whole-gut or colonic transit using radio-opaque markers, and anorectal function testing using a catheter with a balloon. In specialized centers, a few more techniques have been used to some extent: combined impedance and pH monitoring for gastroesophageal reflux, small bowel manometry, satiety drinking tests, breath tests for orocecal transit, scintigraphic colon transit, and defecating proctography. Currently available techniques are reasonably good at detecting well-defined cases of dysmotility (achalasia, gastroesophageal reflux, gastroparesis, pseudo-obstruction, and slow transit constipation). Three of these are actually diagnosed from physiologic parameters: (1) achalasia by absent relaxation of the lower esophageal sphincter (for further details see Chapter 9), (2) gastroparesis by delayed emptying of the stomach, and (3) slow transit constipation by delayed transit through the colon. The diagnosis of gastroesophageal reflux disease can be made from endoscopic findings of erosive esophagitis but also from typical symptoms (heartburn and acid regurgitation) in combination with symptom improvement after antacid or antisecretory medication, whereas 24-hour pH monitoring, impedance, and manometry are seldom used in routine diagnostic work. Pseudo-obstruction is diagnosed on the basis of clinical history (subocclusive events), findings on abdominal roentgenograms (dilated bowel and air/fluid levels), and exclusion of a mechanical cause for obstruction (see Chapter 7). Physiological measurements, such as small bowel manometry, can possibly be used for screening purposes or for differentiation between myopathic and neuropathic types of pseudo-obstruction.[16] The latter, however, remains an issue primarily for the pathologist, if full-thickness bowel tissue can be obtained.[17]

The detection of less well-defined cases of dysmotility is more difficult either because no firm definition exists in terms of motor disturbances or because methods for their detection are lacking. If a patient has alternating diarrhea and constipation, one can hypothesize that these symptoms result from intestinal dysmotility. It is, however, very difficult to prove dysmotility in such a patient using currently available techniques (small bowel transit, small bowel manometry, and colon transit). Even so, because one goal of the Rome process has been to better understand the underlying pathophysiology, groups of patients with FGIDs that no longer are purely without objective findings have been identified. This creates a basis for discussing if dysmotility-associated FGIDs should be defined and if such definitions are useful from a clinical or research point of view?

THE UTILITY OF PHYSIOLOGY-BASED DIAGNOSIS

A diagnosis is, in the ideal situation, the assignment of a patient's complaints to a category that links symptoms with a pathological process and, in some cases, with a specific cause.[18] The classification of patients and their complaints into diagnostic categories is most useful if the diagnosis facilitates an understanding of the nature and causation of the complaints and aids therapeutic or prognostic decision making. The diagnosis of a functional disorder partly helps us in this respect by defining a benign prognosis and some therapeutic options worth trying. It also helps us avoid things not to do, like unnecessary and potentially harmful diagnostic investigations. A major drawback is that our understanding of disease mechanisms is not much enhanced by symptom-based diagnosis, and it is questionable if the symptom-based approach can identify diagnoses with similar etiology, pathogenesis, or pathophysiology.

As an alternative to the Rome process, an international working team presented a pragmatic view on physiology-based diagnosis for the 2002 World Congresses of Gastroenterology in Bangkok.[19] The Bangkok classification divides motility disorders into well-defined entities, entities with a variable dysfunction-symptom relationship, and questionable entities. The well-defined entities in the esophagus comprised gastroesophageal reflux disease, achalasia, and esophageal spasm. Only the diagnosis of dumping syndrome qualified as a well-defined gastric motility disorder and intestinal pseudo-obstruction as a well-defined small bowel motility disorder. Finally, megacolon, Hirschsprung's disease, and slow-transit constipation were classified as diagnoses with a firm relationship between disordered colorectal motility and symptoms.

Few, if any, patients who currently are labeled as FGIDs would receive a physiology-based diagnosis among the well-defined entities of the Bangkok classification but a fair proportion might qualify for entities with a variable dysfunction-symptom relationship. These include gastroparesis, gastric dysrelaxation, sphincter of Oddi dyskinesia, the new diagnostic entity, enteric dysmotility, and fecal incontinence.[19] Several studies have found that 20% to 30% of patients with functional dyspepsia have delayed gastric emptying, thus qualifying for the diagnosis of gastroparesis.[20–23] However, a significant proportion of patients with functional dyspepsia (27%–43%) exhibit an increased rate of emptying, in particular, during the early postprandial phase,[24,25] and about 40% of patients with functional dyspepsia may have gastric dysrelaxation.[26,27] The relation of these pathophysiologic findings to symptoms is weak and inconsistent between studies, but impaired gastric accommodation may be associated with early satiation[28] and delayed gastric emptying with postprandial fullness, nausea, and vomiting.[29] Recently, a large study assessing colon transit by scintigraphy in a cohort of patients with functional constipation and constipation-predominant IBS, concluded that an underlying motor disorder could be found in about 30%.[30] As in functional dyspepsia, a lack of meaningful associations between colon transit and gastrointestinal symptoms other than the stool habits, particularly stool consistency,[31–33] have been hard to find and have not been extensively investigated. Even more problematic is the observation that about one quarter of patients with IBS change their predominant bowel pattern, at least once within a year.[34]

A new entity with a variable dysfunction-symptom relationship that seems to make a difference in prognostic and therapeutic decision making is enteric dysmotility. The increased use of small bowel motility testing in patients with bowel symptoms has made it clear that there exist patients who have disturbances of small bowel motor activity that are characteristic of intestinal pseudo-obstruction but that lack the radiologic features of this diagnosis. Such patients may represent a transitional state between the severe end of the spectrum of functional bowel disorders and pseudo-obstruction or a previously unrecognized subgroup of patients with FGID. The latter is supported by the finding of abnormal motor patterns in 39% of patients with IBS.[35] Patients with enteric dysmotility have a better prognosis and less need for parenteral nutrition than those with intestinal pseudo-obstruction.[16] The meaningfulness of distinguishing enteric dysmotility from IBS remains to be shown.

ADVANCES IN MOTILITY MEASUREMENT

The routine method for esophageal manometry with a water-perfused catheter is now being replaced by high-resolution manometry using catheters with closely spaced solid-state transducers and computer programs that improve graphic presentation of data (see Chapter 9). The pressure profiles of the esophagus and the upper and lower sphincter areas are much easier to interpret both visually and algorithmically by the computerized systems. The high-resolution technique enables us to define 3 subtypes of achalasia based on esophagogastric junction pressures, axial esophagogastric junction movement, and maximal esophageal pressurization.[36] This subclassification has more than academic interest because it may predict treatment outcomes. Type II achalasia with signs of remaining esophageal peristaltic activity responds best to all available treatment options, whereas type III with spastic contraction is a strong negative predictor of treatment response.[37,38]

The high-resolution technique has also been applied to the study of anorectal function.[39] Water-perfused anorectal manometry has previously been done with the patient in the left lateral decubitus position. It is possible, but yet not shown, that the high-resolution technique will facilitate testing of anorectal function with the patient in a more physiologic position.[40]

Fiber optic high-resolution manometry of the colon has recently been developed.[41] This technique certainly holds promise for improving our understanding of colonic motor activity in health and disease. Perhaps this technique can be applied to the study of small bowel motor activity, where there is also room for improvement of our understanding.

Many of the techniques used in gastrointestinal physiology testing today can only be applied under conditions that do not resemble normal activities of daily life. Technological advances have created the opportunity to use ingestible capsules that can measure total and segmental gastrointestinal transit without the use of radiation. The wireless motility capsule measures pressure, pH, and temperature simultaneously and makes it possible to calculate oro-anal transit, gastric residence time, small bowel transit, and colon transit with a single investigation. The characteristic increase in pH from the stomach to the duodenum identifies when the capsule leaves the stomach, and a sudden fall of 1 pH unit marks the entrance into the cecal area. Expulsion is marked by a decrease in temperature when the capsule leaves the body. The wireless motility capsule seems to perform as well as scintigraphy regarding gastric emptying[42,43] and as well as scintigraphy[43] and radio-opaque markers[44] for whole gut and colonic transit. As with many new methods, the cost is considerable, and, as an interesting alternative, the capsule used in capsule endoscopy has been used to detect gut wall activity; these signals translated into motor activity using computer vision technology.[45]

DYSMOTILITY IN FUNCTIONAL DISORDERS

It is obvious from research findings during the last 2 decades that physiologic abnormalities exist in a fair proportion of patients that are labeled functional gastrointestinal disorders. We don't think there is any contradiction between a classification based on symptoms, such as the Rome criteria, and a physiology-based system such as the Bangkok classification. It is also clear that few patients with a symptom-based diagnosis will be shown to suffer from a well-defined motility disorder. The overlap between the 2 classification systems is mainly among entities with a variable dysfunction-symptom relationship. Physiologic findings may well help physicians and patients understand why certain symptoms occur. However, therapeutic implications of physiology-based diagnosis are still uncertain.

Therapeutic interventions aimed at correcting a physiologic abnormality do not necessarily lead to improvement of symptoms. This was shown by several attempts to improve gastric emptying among patients with functional dyspepsia and delayed gastric emptying.[46] On the other hand, tegaserod, a pharmacologic agent with well-defined prokinetic effects in the gastrointestinal tract, was shown to be efficacious for the improvement of stool consistency and moderately effective in the reduction of symptoms like abdominal pain, discomfort, and bloating in constipated IBS patients.[47] Therapeutic trials with inclusion criteria involving both physiologic and functional vectors in the definition of diagnostic subgroups would probably move our knowledge forward by merging rather than separating functional and dysmotility groups. A recent example is the evaluation of linaclotide for constipation. Stool consistency judged by the Bristol Stool Form scale[48] as 6 (mushy) more than once, and 7 (watery) at any time during screening, excluded patients from study participation.[49] Assessing stool consistency is admittedly not equivalent to physiologic measurement, but stool consistency correlates well with colonic transit.[31]

SUMMARY

Taken together, the above examples indicate that physiology-based diagnosis has a substantial overlap with symptom-based diagnosis. Neither symptomatic treatment nor therapy aimed at restoring normal physiology has had much success. It is still uncertain if measurement of physiologic parameters facilitates the doctor-patient relationship, whether results are abnormal or normal. However, the addition of physiology parameters to the evaluation of therapeutic interventions aimed at symptom reduction in FGIDs can possibly facilitate the identification of subgroups with a higher probability of treatment success. Unfortunately, our experience from clinical trials in this area is that physiology testing usually disappears as a new drug moves from phase II to phase III trials. In the ideal situation, the development of measurement methods with better availability and standardization, like different ingestible capsules, will help us to merge physiology and symptoms regarding both diagnosis and treatment evaluation.

REFERENCES

1. Longstreth GF, Thompson WG, Chey WD, et al. Functional bowel disorders. Gastroenterology 2006;130(5):1480–91.
2. Drossman DA. The functional gastrointestinal disorders and the Rome III process. Gastroenterology 2006;130(5):1377–90.

3. Spiegel BM, Farid M, Esrailian E, et al. Is irritable bowel syndrome a diagnosis of exclusion? A survey of primary care providers, gastroenterologists, and IBS experts. Am J Gastroenterol 2010;105(4):848–58.
4. Agréus L, Svärdsudd K, Nyrén O, et al. Irritable bowel syndrome and dyspepsia in the general population: overlap and lack of stability over time. Gastroenterology 1995; 109(3):671–80.
5. Agréus L, Svärdsudd K, Talley NJ, et al. Natural history of gastroesophageal reflux disease and functional abdominal disorders: a population-based study. Am J Gastroenterol 2001;96(10):2905–14.
6. Harvey RF, Hinton RA, Gunary RM, et al. Individual and group hypnotherapy in treatment of refractory irritable bowel syndrome. Lancet 1989;1(8635):424–5.
7. Owens DM, Nelson DK, Talley NJ. The irritable bowel syndrome: long-term prognosis and the physician-patient interaction. Ann Intern Med 1995;122(2):107–12.
8. Svendsen JH, Munck LK, Andersen JR. Irritable bowel syndrome—prognosis and diagnostic safety. A 5-year follow-up study. Scand J Gastroenterol 1985;20(4): 415–18.
9. Koloski NA, Talley NJ, Boyce PM. Predictors of health care seeking for irritable bowel syndrome and nonulcer dyspepsia: a critical review of the literature on symptom and psychosocial factors. Am J Gastroenterol 2001;96(5):1340–49.
10. Kaptchuk TJ, Kelley JM, Conboy LA, et al. Components of placebo effect: randomised controlled trial in patients with irritable bowel syndrome. BMJ 2008; 336(7651):999–1003.
11. Patel SM, Stason WB, Legedza A, et al. The placebo effect in irritable bowel syndrome trials: a meta-analysis. Neurogastroenterol Motil 2005;17(3):332–40.
12. Parkman HP, Hasler WL, Barnett JL, et al. Electrogastrography: a document prepared by the gastric section of the American Motility Society Clinical GI Motility Testing Task Force. Neurogastroenterol Motil 2003;15(2):89–102.
13. Gilja OH, Detmer PR, Jong JM, et al. Intragastric distribution and gastric emptying assessed by three-dimensional ultrasonography. Gastroenterology 1997;113(1): 38–49.
14. Clemens CH, Samsom M, Van Berge Henegouwen GP, et al. Abnormalities of left colonic motility in ambulant nonconstipated patients with irritable bowel syndrome. Dig Dis Sci 2003;48(1):74–82.
15. Herbst F, Kamm MA, Morris GP, et al. Gastrointestinal transit and prolonged ambulatory colonic motility in health and faecal incontinence. Gut 1997;41(3):381–9.
16. Lindberg G, Iwarzon M, Törnblom H. Clinical features and long-term survival in chronic intestinal pseudo-obstruction and enteric dysmotility. Scand J Gastroenterol 2009; 44(6):692–99.
17. Lindberg G, Törnblom H, Iwarzon M, et al. Full-thickness biopsy findings in chronic intestinal pseudo-obstruction and enteric dysmotility. Gut 2009;58(8):1084–90.
18. McWhinney IR. A textbook of family medicine. New York: Oxford University Press; 1989.
19. Wingate D, Hongo M, Kellow J, et al. Disorders of gastrointestinal motility: towards a new classification. J Gastroenterol Hepatol 2002;17(Suppl):S1–14.
20. Bisschops R, Karamanolis G, Arts J, et al. Relationship between symptoms and ingestion of a meal in functional dyspepsia. Gut 2008;57(11):1495–1503.
21. Maes BD, Ghoos YF, Hiele MI, et al. Gastric emptying rate of solids in patients with nonulcer dyspepsia. Dig Dis Sci 1997;42(6):1158–62.
22. Perri F, Clemente R, Festa V, et al. Patterns of symptoms in functional dyspepsia: role of Helicobacter pylori infection and delayed gastric emptying. Am J Gastroenterol 1998;93(11):2082–8.

23. Stanghellini V, Tosetti C, Paternico A, et al. Risk indicators of delayed gastric emptying of solids in patients with functional dyspepsia. Gastroenterology 1996; 110(4):1036–42.
24. Delgado-Aros S, Camilleri M, Cremonini F, et al. Contributions of gastric volumes and gastric emptying to meal size and postmeal symptoms in functional dyspepsia. Gastroenterology 2004;127(6):1685–94.
25. Zai H, Kusano M. Investigation of gastric emptying disorders in patients with functional dyspepsia reveals impaired inhibitory gastric emptying regulation in the early postcibal period. Digestion 2009;79 (Suppl 1):13–18.
26. Bredenoord AJ, Chial HJ, Camilleri M, et al. Gastric accommodation and emptying in evaluation of patients with upper gastrointestinal symptoms. Clin Gastroenterol Hepatol 2003;1(4):264–72.
27. Tack J, Caenepeel P, Piessevaux H, et al. Assessment of meal induced gastric accommodation by a satiety drinking test in health and in severe functional dyspepsia. Gut 2003;52(9):1271–7.
28. Tack J, Piessevaux H, Coulie B, et al. Role of impaired gastric accommodation to a meal in functional dyspepsia. Gastroenterology 1998;115(6):1346–52.
29. Sarnelli G, Caenepeel P, Geypens B, et al. Symptoms associated with impaired gastric emptying of solids and liquids in functional dyspepsia. Am J Gastroenterol 2003;98(4):783–8.
30. Manabe N, Wong BS, Camilleri M, et al. Lower functional gastrointestinal disorders: evidence of abnormal colonic transit in a 287 patient cohort. Neurogastroenterol Motil 2010;22(3):293–e282.
31. Degen LP, Phillips SF. How well does stool form reflect colonic transit? Gut 1996; 39(1):109–13.
32. O'Donnell LJ, Virjee J, Heaton KW. Detection of pseudodiarrhoea by simple clinical assessment of intestinal transit rate. BMJ 1990;300(6722):439–40.
33. Saad RJ, Rao SS, Koch KL, et al. Do stool form and frequency correlate with whole-gut and colonic transit? Results from a multicenter study in constipated individuals and healthy controls. Am J Gastroenterol 2010;105(2):403–11.
34. Drossman DA, Morris CB, Hu Y, et al. A prospective assessment of bowel habit in irritable bowel syndrome in women: defining an alternator. Gastroenterology 2005; 128(3):580–9.
35. Simrén M, Castedal M, Svedlund J, et al. Abnormal propagation pattern of duodenal pressure waves in the irritable bowel syndrome (IBS). Dig Dis Sci 2000;45(11):2151–61.
36. Pandolfino JE, Ghosh SK, Rice J, et al. Classifying esophageal motility by pressure topography characteristics: a study of 400 patients and 75 controls. Am J Gastroenterol 2008;103(1):27–37.
37. Pandolfino JE, Kwiatek MA, Nealis T, et al. Achalasia: a new clinically relevant classification by high-resolution manometry. Gastroenterology 2008;135(5): 1526–33.
38. Pratap N, Kalapala R, Darisetty S, et al. Achalasia cardia subtyping by high-resolution manometry predicts the therapeutic outcome of pneumatic balloon dilatation. J Neurogastroenterol Motil 2011;17(1):48–53.
39. Jones MP, Post J, Crowell MD. High-resolution manometry in the evaluation of anorectal disorders: a simultaneous comparison with water-perfused manometry. Am J Gastroenterol 2007;102(4):850–5.
40. Rao SS, Kavlock R, Rao S. Influence of body position and stool characteristics on defecation in humans. Am J Gastroenterol 2006;101(12):2790–6.

41. Arkwright JW, Underhill ID, Maunder SA, et al. Design of a high-sensor count fibre optic manometry catheter for in-vivo colonic diagnostics. Opt Express 2009;17(25): 22423–31.
42. Kuo B, McCallum RW, Koch KL, et al. Comparison of gastric emptying of a nondigestible capsule to a radio-labelled meal in healthy and gastroparetic subjects. Aliment Pharmacol Ther 2008;27(2):186–96.
43. Maqbool S, Parkman HP, Friedenberg FK. Wireless capsule motility: comparison of the SmartPill GI monitoring system with scintigraphy for measuring whole gut transit. Dig Dis Sci 2009;54(10):2167–74.
44. Rao SS, Kuo B, McCallum RW, et al. Investigation of colonic and whole-gut transit with wireless motility capsule and radiopaque markers in constipation. Clin Gastroenterol Hepatol 2009;7(5):537–44.
45. Malagelada C, De Iorio F, Azpiroz F, et al. New insight into intestinal motor function via noninvasive endoluminal image analysis. Gastroenterology 2008;135(4):1155–62.
46. Sanger GJ, Alpers DH. Development of drugs for gastrointestinal motor disorders: translating science to clinical need. Neurogastroenterol Motil 2008;20(3):177–84.
47. Evans BW, Clark WK, Moore DJ, et al. Tegaserod for the treatment of irritable bowel syndrome and chronic constipation. Cochrane Database Syst Rev 2007(4): CD003960.
48. Lewis SJ, Heaton KW. Stool form scale as a useful guide to intestinal transit time. Scand J Gastroenterol 1997;32(9):920–4.
49. Lembo AJ, Kurtz CB, Macdougall JE, et al. Efficacy of linaclotide for patients with chronic constipation. Gastroenterology 2010;138(3):886–95.e1.

Gastrointestinal Dysmotility: Clinical Consequences and Management of the Critically Ill Patient

Marianne J. Chapman, BMBS, PhD, FCICM[a,b,*],
Nam Q. Nguyen, MBBS (Hons), PhD, FRACP[c,d],
Adam M. Deane, MBBS, FRACP, FCICM[a,b]

KEYWORDS

• Critical illness • Gastrointestinal motility • Gastric emptying
• Nutrient absorption • Prokinetic • Enteral feeding

Gastrointestinal motility can be markedly deranged in critical illness.[1] This can have a number of important clinical sequelae—the most obvious of which is impaired delivery of enteral nutrition, which can result in malnutrition, if not recognized and treated. Impaired gastric emptying and lower esophageal sphincter function may allow reflux of gastric contents into the esophagus during enteral feeding, especially in the recumbent position. This situation, combined with the loss of normal airway reflexes in the sedated and sometimes paralyzed patient, results in aspiration, which can be subclinical and therefore unrecognized, impairing respiratory function and predisposing to ventilator-associated pneumonia. Another proposed consequence of gastrointestinal dysmotility in the critically ill is intestinal stasis with bacterial overgrowth, potentially leading to bacterial translocation and nosocomial sepsis. However, this has never been conclusively demonstrated in humans.

This work was supported by grants from the National Health and Medical Research Council and the Australian and New Zealand College of Anaesthesia.
The authors have nothing to disclose.
[a] Department of Critical Care Services, Royal Adelaide Hospital, North Terrace, Adelaide, South Australia 5000, Australia
[b] Discipline of Acute Care Medicine, School of Medicine, University of Adelaide, Adelaide, South Australia, Australia
[c] Department of Gastroenterology and Hepatology, Royal Adelaide Hospital, North Terrace, Adelaide, South Australia 5000, Australia
[d] Discipline of Medicine, School of Medicine, University of Adelaide, Adelaide, South Australia, Australia
* Corresponding author.
E-mail address: Marianne.chapman@health.sa.gov.au

Gastroenterol Clin N Am 40 (2011) 725–739
doi:10.1016/j.gtc.2011.09.003
gastro.theclinics.com
0889-8553/11/$ – see front matter

ESOPHAGEAL MOTILITY

The gastroesophageal sphincter has reduced activity in critical illness, which can have important clinical consequences. Basal lower esophageal pressures are reduced when compared to health and acid reflux occurs frequently during fasting and gastric feeding. Furthermore, reflux contents remain in the esophagus for prolonged periods as clearance is markedly impaired. Most reflux episodes occur because of very low or, in some cases, absent lower esophageal sphincter pressures.[2,3] Reflux episodes are also associated with straining and coughing on the endotracheal tube.[2]

GASTRIC MOTILITY

Gastric motility can be markedly abnormal in critical illness resulting in slow gastric emptying and reduced ability to tolerate nasogastric delivery of nutrients. The stomach may be functionally divided into proximal and distal parts and, in order to achieve optimal gastric emptying, the motility of these regions needs to be coordinated. During critical illness, not only is the motility of each region disturbed, but also the motor integration between the proximal and distal stomach is disrupted.[4]

Fundal tone is important for normal gastric emptying of liquid nutrient[5] and, is, therefore, likely to be fundamental to the gastric emptying of liquid formulae in the critically ill patient. In health, proximal gastric relaxation occurs in response to the presence of duodenal nutrient. In critical illness, accommodation of the proximal stomach in response to small intestinal nutrient is delayed and there is increased retention in the proximal stomach.[6] These abnormal patterns of motility are likely to result in delayed distribution of ingesta to the distal stomach, which will slow gastric emptying and, potentially, increase the risk of gastroesophageal reflux.

Reduced fasting antral motility, which is characterized by the absence, or reduction, of the antral component of phase 3 of the interdigestive migrating motor complex (MMC), occurs in critical illness and is associated with slow gastric emptying.[1,7] An absence or reduction of antral phase 3 activity may predispose to colonization of the stomach with microbial pathogens. In critically ill patients this could have serious consequences, as it may be a precursor of ventilator-associated pneumonia.[8]

In health, the rate of gastric emptying is directly related to antral activity[9] and, hence, delayed gastric emptying may be associated with weak and/or disordered antroduodenal contractions.[10] Reduced postprandial antral activity has been reported in critically ill patients.[1,7] Furthermore, erythromycin markedly increases antral wave activity and accelerates gastric emptying in this group.[11,12] Thus, a direct relationship between gastric emptying and antral activity in the critically ill has been established.

Pyloric activity (phasic and tonic) is integral to the regulation of gastric emptying. Both increased basal pyloric pressure and more frequent phasic contractions have been demonstrated in critically ill patients, and these abnormalities have been shown to correlate with slow gastric emptying (**Fig. 1**).[1]

SMALL INTESTINAL MOTILITY

Slow gastric emptying will delay delivery of nutrient to the small intestine resulting in a reduced rate of nutrient absorption. Small intestinal motility is also impaired in critical illness, which has the potential to further reduce nutrient absorption and contribute to the malnutrition of critical illness. Abnormalities in MMC activity may be characterized by changes in the proportion of time spent in the 3 phases, the coordination of contractions during the phases, and/or the direction of migration of phase III activity. Furthermore, persistence of MMC activity during feeding is

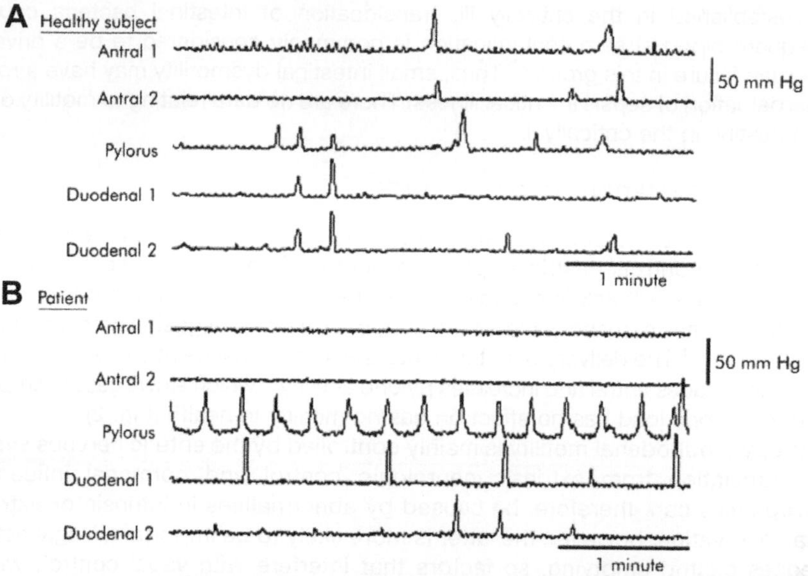

Fig. 1. Recording of pressure waves in antral, pyloric, and duodenal channels in a healthy subject *(A)* and a critically ill patient *(B)* during an intraduodenal infusion of liquid nutrient (1 kcal/min). The reduction in antral activity and marked increase in isolated pyloric pressure wave frequency observed in the critically ill patient are motor patterns which will slow gastric emptying. (*From* Chapman M, Fraser R, Vozzo R, et al. Antro-pyloro-duodenal motor responses to gastric and duodenal nutrient in critically ill patients. Gut 2005;54:1384–90; with permission.)

considered pathologic, although its implications are unclear. The relationship between the frequency of phase III activity and small intestinal transit is uncertain. Both more frequent MMC activity and delayed transit have been demonstrated following the administration of opioids[13] and postoperatively.[14–16] These are relevant to critical illness.

In critical illness, during fasting, the number of contractions and the occurrence of activity fronts in the duodenum (proximal and distal) are comparable to health.[17] Although the duration of the duodenal MMC is also similar, the relative contribution of the quiescent period (phase 1) to the total cycle length is increased and that of phase 2 activity reduced.[7,16] The activity fronts are also abnormal in character with retrograde or stationary propagation.[1,7,16–18] Furthermore, fasting activity has been reported to persist in some critically ill patients during feeding,[18–22] and, while the clinical implications of this are uncertain, data suggest that this may be associated with reduced absorption in patients following major abdominal surgery.[23]

Small intestinal transit has rarely been evaluated in the critically ill, but it does not appear to be substantially faster than in health.[24,25] This is relevant as rapid transit can attenuate absorption.[24] In the critically ill, no relationship between transit and nutrient absorption has been demonstrated.[24]

The normal intestinal microbiota stimulates the initiation and aboral migration of physiologic phase III activity and, conversely, loss of normal MMC activity is associated with small intestinal bacterial overgrowth in health.[26–28] The microbiota in critical illness is unlikely to be normal but the effect of any abnormality on intestinal motility is unclear. While this relationship between motility and overgrowth has not been established in the critically ill, translocation of intestinal bacteria causing subsequent blood stream contamination is commonly considered to be a driver of multiorgan failure in this group.[29] Thus, small intestinal dysmotility may have a role in the perpetuation of sepsis in critical illness. There are no data relating to motility of the large intestine in the critically ill.

CONTROL OF GASTROINTESTINAL MOTILITY

In health, nutrient interacts with small intestinal receptors and, via neurohumoral mechanisms, controls gastric emptying at a rate of about 2 to 3 kcal/min.[30] This small intestinal feedback is exaggerated in the critically ill and appears to be the principal mechanism responsible for the abnormal slowing of gastric emptying during enteral feeding.[1] The delivery of nutrient into the small intestine at a rate of as little as 1 kcal/min reduces antral and increases pyloric activity,[1] which slows gastric empting; this same caloric load has no effect on gastric motility in health (**Fig. 2**).

Antropyloroduodenal motility is mainly controlled by the enteric nervous system with modulation from extrinsic neurologic control and hormonal influences. Gastroparesis can, therefore, be caused by abnormalities in intrinsic or extrinsic neural innervation; however, the latter is more likely to be important. Vagal activity increases gastric emptying, so factors that interfere with vagal control, will be inhibitory. Vagal neuropathy is considered an important mediator of gastroparesis in ambulant diabetics[31] and could be a factor in critical illness. The vagus is also important in the control of fasting motility. Abolition of fasting motility by food intake requires an intact vagus[32] and, therefore, persistence of MMC activity during feeding suggests abnormal extrinsic neural control.[33] The failure of abolition of fasting motility patterns by feeding in some critically ill patients may be a result of reduced vagal activity.

Sympathetic activity inhibits gastrointestinal motility and sympathetic overactivity is a feature of critical illness. Therefore, sympathetic neural stimulation may have a role in gastrointestinal dysmotility in the critically ill.

Numerous hormones are involved in the regulation of gastrointestinal motility (**Fig. 3**). Cholecystokinin (CCK) is an important humoral mediator of the enterogastric feedback response in health, and also appears to have a role in feeding intolerance and delayed gastric emptying in the critically ill.[34–41] Reduced fasting ghrelin concentrations and elevated fasting and postprandial peptide YY (PYY) levels have been measured in the critically ill[42,43]; however, the relative contributions of the different gastrointestinal hormones to the control of gastric emptying in the critically ill have not been studied.

The hormone that appears to be most important in the control of the MMC in health is motilin. Intravenous administration of motilin,[44] or 1 to 3 mg/kg/h of the motilin agonist erythromycin,[45] induces "phase III–like" activity in the antroduodenal region. Motilin levels peak during MMC activity. The effect of erythromycin on MMC activity is highly relevant to critically ill patients as erythromycin is used as a prokinetic. While fasting plasma motilin concentrations were recently shown to be similar in critically ill patients and healthy subjects, plasma motilin concentrations were significantly higher in the patients during nutrient infusion. In addition, there was an inverse relationship between the peak increase in plasma motilin concentrations and the peak change in proximal gastric volume induced by duodenal nutrient stimulation in critically ill subjects. These findings may explain the persistence in interdigestive gastrointestinal contractile activity and the impaired proximal gastric relaxation during enteral feeding in these patients.[46]

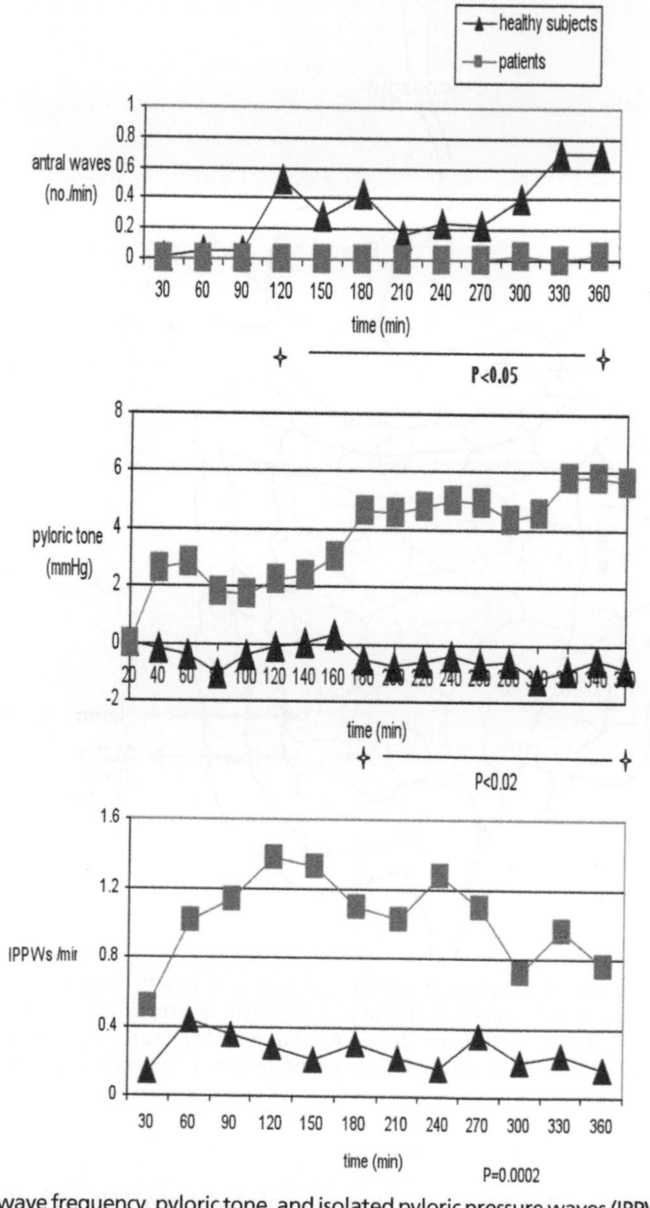

Fig. 2. Antral wave frequency, pyloric tone, and isolated pyloric pressure waves (IPPW) frequency over time during duodenal infusion of nutrient at 1 kcal/min in critically ill patients and healthy subjects. (*From* Chapman M, Fraser R, Vozzo R, et al. Antro-pyloro-duodenal motor responses to gastric and duodenal nutrient in critically ill patients. Gut 2005;54:1384–90; with permission.)

CONSEQUENCES OF GASTROINTESTINAL DYSMOTILITY IN THE INTENSIVE CARE UNIT

Gastroesophageal Reflux and Aspiration

Reflux episodes combined with the loss of normal airway reflexes in the sedated and sometimes paralyzed patient results in aspiration,[47] which can lead to impaired

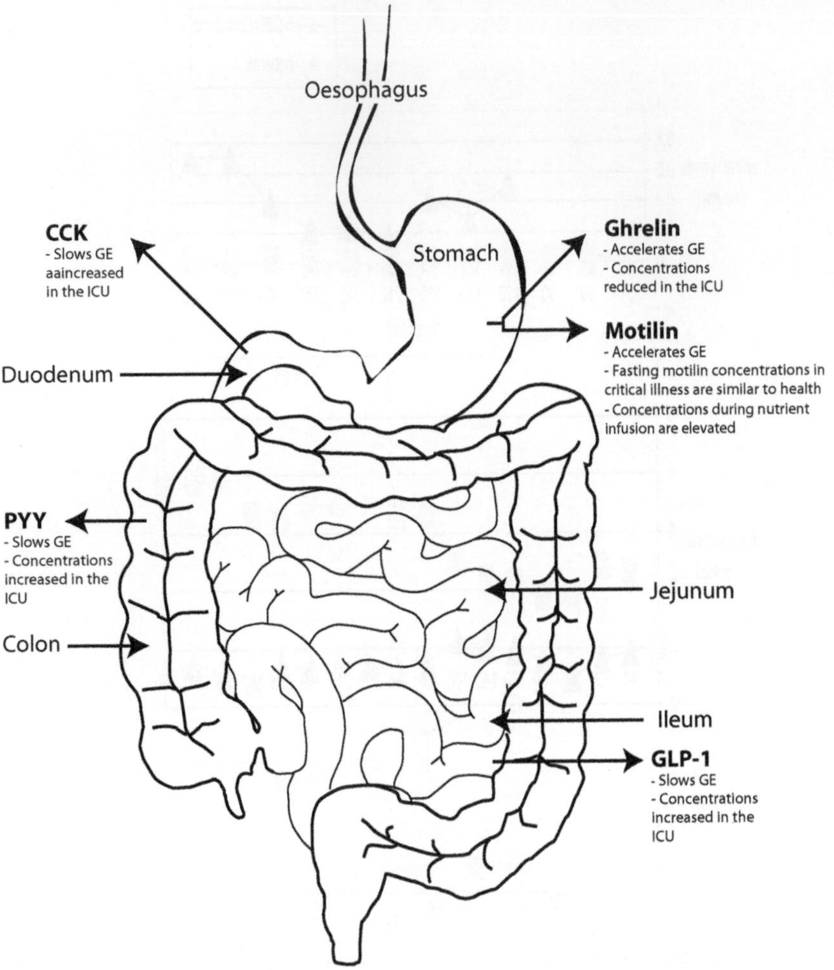

Fig. 3. The effects of hormones on gastric emptying in health and their known fasting concentration in patients admitted to the ICU: CCK (cholecystokinin), GLP-1 (glucagon-like peptide-1), PYY (peptide YY). (*From* Deane A, Chapman MJ, Fraser RJ, Horowitz M. Bench-to-bedside review: The gut as an endocrine organ in the critically ill. Crit Care 2010;14:228; with permission.)

respiratory function. The relationship between gastric dysmotility and reflux is, as yet, unclear but there is some evidence that feeding directly into the small intestine reduces the risk of reflux and nosocomial pneumonia.[48]

Slow Gastric Emptying

Gastric emptying is delayed in about 50% of mechanically ventilated, critically ill patients.[49–52] Gastric emptying can be markedly slowed,[53,54] with about 1 in 5 patients emptying less than 50% of gastric contents at 4 hours.[50] Certain diagnostic groups appear more likely to have slow gastric emptying[50,55] (**Fig. 4**), and delays have been associated with increasing severity of illness.[50] The cause of slow gastric

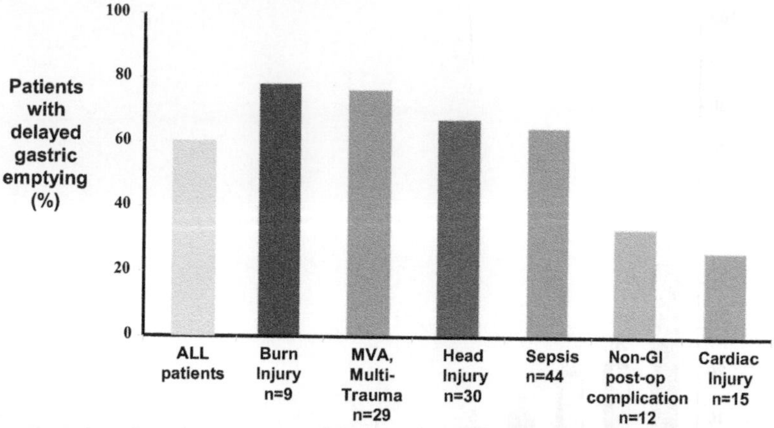

Fig. 4. Impact of admission diagnosis on gastric emptying in 132 mixed mechanically ventilated patients. (*From* Nguyen NQ, Ng MP, Chapman M, Fraser RJ, Holloway RH. The impact of admission diagnosis on gastric emptying in critically ill patients. Crit Care 2007;11:R16; with permission.)

emptying is likely to be multifactorial, with certain parameters having more or less importance in different patients. Additional factors associated with slow gastric emptying in the critically ill include raised intracranial pressure,[56,57] reduced level of consciousness as measured using the Glasgow Coma Scale,[53] time from traumatic brain injury,[53] the height of a spinal cord lesion,[58] increasing age,[52,58] and administration of dopamine.[51] Dopamine, a commonly used inotrope, reduces antral contractions, shortens MMC duration,[21] and slows gastric emptying and orocecal transit time.[59] This is likely to be mediated through central and peripheral effects. Other catecholamines, such as epinephrine, also stimulate beta-adrenergic receptors to slow gastric emptying.[60,61] There are conflicting data in relation to the effects of the administration of opiates[52,56,62] and gender.[52,53] Electrolyte abnormalities such as hyperglycemia, recent surgery, shock, circulating cytokines, or the disease process itself[63] are also likely to contribute. In health, acute elevations in blood glucose concentrations reduce gastroduodenal motility and slow gastric emptying,[64,65] and high blood glucose concentrations occur frequently in the critically ill. We have demonstrated a relationship between hyperglycemia and feed intolerance[66]; however, this may not be causal as it is likely that factors which act to increase blood glucose concentrations, such as severity of illness and catecholamine requirement, may also slow gastric emptying. Interestingly, preexisting diabetes does not appear to be a risk factor for feed intolerance or delayed gastric emptying in critical illness.[67,68]

Feed Intolerance

Intolerance to intragastric nutrition occurs commonly in critical illness. In a recent prospective, observational study in mechanically ventilated, intragastrically fed patients, the prevalence of "feed-intolerance" was approximately 35% (defined as a gastric residual volume of 250 ml or more),[69] and the first episode of feed intolerance occurred early following admission to the ICU[69] (**Fig. 5**). However, the definition of feed intolerance is disputed and the implication of large gastric residual volumes (which are commonly used to define feed tolerance) is unclear. Volumes aspirated from the stomach are affected not only by the rate of gastric emptying[50] but also by

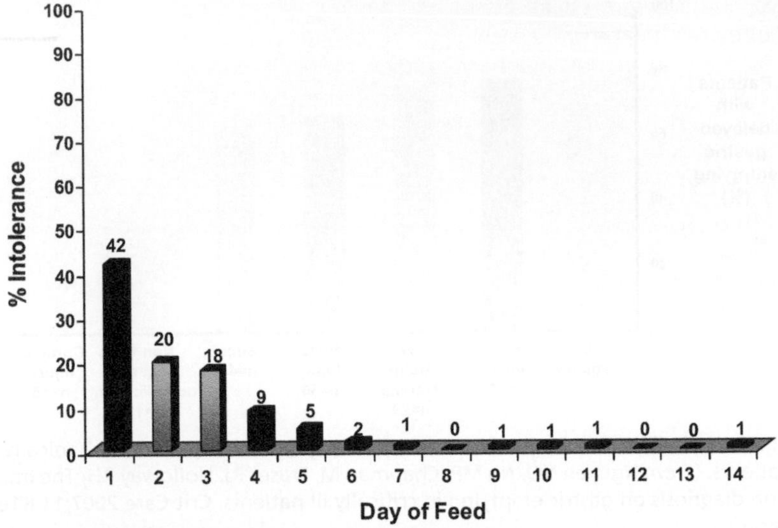

Fig. 5. Timing of the first episode of feed intolerance in patients who failed feeding. Intolerance is defined as gastric residual volume of ≥250 ml.

the rate of feed administration, gastric secretion, and duodenogastric reflux.[70] The course of action that should be taken when a large gastric residual volume is obtained is debated. Currently, the majority of ICUs have protocols for feeding that recommend a change in delivery rate, or the initiation of a prokinetic drug or direct delivery of nutrient into the small intestine, if the gastric residual volume is between 150 and 500 ml.[71] Our data suggest that a cumulative gastric residual volume over the preceding 24 hours of 150 ml or more has a positive predictive value of 0.78 (95% confidence interval [CI], 0.458 to 0.959) and a negative predictive value of 0.69 (95% CI, 0.423 to 0.893) for predicting slow gastric emptying, as subsequently measured by scintigraphy (the gold standard). However, the high rate of esophageal regurgitation and aspiration observed in these patients appears to be independent of gastric residual volume.[71,72] As it is believed to be important to deliver energy goals to ICU patients, it appears unnecessary and inappropriate to change the rate of nutrient administration in response to large gastric volumes. However, as a large gastric residual volume suggests delayed gastric emptying, it may be logical to take action to improve nutrient delivery into the small intestine. This could be achieved by the administration of a prokinetic agent or the delivery of nutrient directly into the small intestine (see later).

Small Intestinal Dysmotility

The clinical significance of abnormal duodenal motility in critical illness remains uncertain. In a small pilot study of fasting patients with severe trauma, the fasting MMC pattern was only present in 50% of the patients, but its presence predicted subsequent successful enteral feeding by jejunostomy (defined by the absence of gastrointestinal symptoms).[22] However, as only 5 patients had fasting MMC activity, this hypothesis needs confirmation in a larger study. The impact of the persistence of fasting motor activity during nutrient administration on gastric emptying and feed tolerance in the critically ill is unclear. Given that the coordination of waves during phase III activity, and the migration of phase III activity may be abnormal in the critically ill, persistent phase III activity may hinder effective nasogastric or jejunal feeding, by reducing small intestinal absorption. Assessing the impact of persistent MMC activity on gastric emptying, the success of feeding, absorption, and the incidence of complications such as diarrhea is relevant to the ICU population, as it may offer the potential for therapeutic intervention.

Nutrient Malabsorption

Nutrient absorption is impaired in the critically ill and this is likely to contribute to the weight loss that occurs with prolonged ICU stay. The distinction between "rate" of absorption, which is affected by the rate of gastric emptying, and "total" absorption, which is influenced primarily by small intestinal mucosal/pancreatic function, is important. Both the rate and extent of glucose absorption are markedly reduced in the critically ill,[73–77] and there is a close relationship between glucose absorption and gastric emptying such that slow gastric empting is associated with a reduced rate of absorption.[73] Furthermore, even when glucose is placed directly into the small intestine, absorption is impaired, confirming that small intestinal factors also play a role.[24,78] Glucose absorption is dependent on a number of factors that include gastric emptying, small intestinal motility, and transit (which influence contact time with the small intestinal mucosa), the presence of pancreatic enzymes, contact surface area (length of intestine, surface villi, enzyme content of brush border, and function of carrier molecules) and the depth of the diffusion barrier of the absorptive epithelium (unstirred layer).[79] No relationship between transit (measured by scintigraphy) and absorption has been demonstrated in critical illness.[24] However, the small intestinal mucosa is frequently abnormal.[80] Delayed initiation of feeding is associated with reduced absorption, suggesting that a period of fasting may exacerbate mucosal damage.[81] More research on the etiology of impaired absorption is awaited. In critically ill patients, nutrient is delivered continuously into the gut. Ideally, delivery to the small intestine should be at a rate where absorption can be maximized while minimizing the possibility of adverse events such as diarrhea.

THERAPEUTIC APPROACHES TO GASTROINTESTINAL DYSMOTILITY IN THE INTENSIVE CARE UNIT

General Management

There are a number of factors in the general management of the ICU patient that can be used to treat and/or prevent gut dysmotility and avoid its sequelae. These include patient posture, which should be at least 30° head up to reduce aspiration and nosocomial pneumonia in the setting of absent gastroesophageal pressure.[47,82] Reduction in the dosage of opiates[62,83] and catecholamines to minimal tolerated levels and avoidance of the use of dopamine[21] will also reduce exogenous causes of delayed gastric emptying. Hyperglycemia may contribute to slow gastric emptying and blood glucose should be controlled. Prolonged fasting may affect gastrointestinal motility,[84] but early initiation of feeding has not been shown to affect subsequent gastric emptying or gastrointestinal hormones[85] but does improve subsequent nutrient absorption.[81]

Prokinetic Agents

Therapeutic measures to modify gastrointestinal dysmotility in critical illness are limited. Gamma-amino butyric acid-B agonists, such as baclofen or lesogaberan, have been shown, in experimental settings, to increase gastroesophageal junctional pressures[86,87] and have the potential to reduce reflux episodes and subsequent complications, but have not been studied in this patient group. Erythromycin and, to a lesser extent, metoclopramide accelerate gastric emptying in the critically ill[11,12,88] and improve the success of nasogastric feeding and calorie delivery.[89] These agents appear more potent when they are used in combination,[90] as tachyphylaxis is reduced.[90] Furthermore, there is an inverse relationship between plasma erythromycin concentrations and its durability of prokinetic action, where feed-intolerant patients who have lower plasma erythromycin concentrations have a longer response to therapy.[91] Along with vitro studies that show motilin receptor expression is down-regulated via internalization or endocytosis of the receptors after repeated exposure of muscle strips to high concentrations of erythromycin,[92,93] these findings provide not only potential insights into the mechanisms of action but also therapeutic strategies to overcome erythromycin related tachyphylaxis in critically ill patients. As the effect of 70 mg erythromycin on gastric emptying is similar to that of a 200 mg dose in critically ill patients, one strategy to minimize tachyphylaxis is to reduce the dose to 70 mg twice daily.[12] Alternatively, measuring plasma concentrations of erythromycin after the first dose can be used to adjust the subsequent dosing given that a trough plasma erythromycin level of 0.5 mg/L or greater had 83% sensitivity and 72% specificity ($P = 0.007$, AUC = 0.80) in predicting loss of response to erythromycin over 7 days.[91] This warrants further study.

Other novel gastrokinetic drugs, such as nonantibiotic motilin agonists, ghrelin agonists, or CCK antagonists (eg, dexloxiglumide), could be of interest but are yet to be investigated.[94]

Postpyloric Feeding

Delivery of nutrient directly into the small intestine using a small intestinal feeding catheter is frequently instituted by intensivists when gastric feeding in combination with prokinetic therapy has failed. Newer techniques for small intestinal tube insertion facilitate more convenient and rapid placement without the need for endoscopy.[95,96] However, small intestinal feeding has not been consistently shown to increase energy delivery or improve clinical outcomes[97,98] and recent preliminary data suggest that nutrient absorption may not be increased when nutrients are placed directly into the small intestine.[24,99]

SUMMARY

Gastrointestinal dysmotility is a common feature of critical illness, with a number of significant implications that include malnutrition secondary to reduced feed tolerance and absorption, reflux and aspiration resulting in reduced lung function and ventilator-associated pneumonia, bacterial overgrowth and possible translocation causing nosocomial sepsis. Prokinetic agent administration can improve gastric emptying and caloric delivery, but its effect on nutrient absorption and clinical outcomes is, as yet, unclear. Postpyloric delivery of nutrition has not yet been demonstrated to increase caloric intake or improve clinical outcomes.

REFERENCES

1. Chapman M, Fraser R, Vozzo R, et al. Antro-pyloro-duodenal motor responses to gastric and duodenal nutrient in critically ill patients. Gut 2005;54:1384–90.
2. Nind G, Chen WH, Protheroe R, et al. Mechanisms of gastroesophageal reflux in critically ill mechanically ventilated patients. Gastroenterology 2005;128:600–6.
3. Wilmer A, Tack J, Frans E, et al. Duodenogastroesophageal reflux and esophageal mucosal injury in mechanically ventilated patients. Gastroenterology 1999;116:1293–9.

4. Nguyen NQ, Fraser RJ, Bryant LK, Chapman M, Holloway RH. Diminished functional association between proximal and distal gastric motility in critically ill patients. Intensive Care Med 2008.
5. Kelly KA. Gastric emptying of liquids and solids: roles of proximal and distal stomach. Am J Physiol 1980;239:G71–6.
6. Nguyen NQ, Fraser RJ, Chapman M, et al. Proximal gastric response to small intestinal nutrients is abnormal in mechanically ventilated critically ill patients. World J Gastroenterol 2006;12:4383–8.
7. Dive A, Moulart M, Jonard P, Jamart J, Mahieu P. Gastroduodenal motility in mechanically ventilated critically ill patients: a manometric study. Crit Care Med 1994;22:441–7.
8. Inglis TJ, Sherratt MJ, Sproat LJ, Gibson JS, Hawkey PM. Gastroduodenal dysfunction and bacterial colonisation of the ventilated lung. Lancet 1993;341:911–3.
9. Houghton LA, Read NW, Heddle R, et al. Relationship of the motor activity of the antrum, pylorus, and duodenum to gastric emptying of a solid-liquid mixed meal. Gastroenterology 1988;94:1285–91.
10. Fone DR, Horowitz M, Maddox A, Akkermans LM, Read NW, Dent J. Gastroduodenal motility during the delayed gastric emptying induced by cold stress. Gastroenterology 1990;98(5 Pt 1):1155–61.
11. Dive A, Miesse C, Galanti L, et al. Effect of erythromycin on gastric motility in mechanically ventilated critically ill patients: a double-blind, randomized, placebo-controlled study. Crit Care Med 1995;23:1356–62.
12. Ritz MA, Chapman MJ, Fraser RJ, et al. Erythromycin dose of 70 mg accelerates gastric emptying as effectively as 200 mg in the critically ill. Intensive Care Med 2005;31:949–54.
13. Powell DW. Muscle or mucosa: the site of action of antidiarrheal opiates? Gastroenterology 1981;80:406–8.
14. Noer T. Roentgenological transit time through the small intestine in the immediate postoperative period. Acta Chir Scand 1968;134:577–80.
15. Benson MJ, Roberts JP, Wingate DL, et al. Small bowel motility following major intra-abdominal surgery: the effects of opiates and rectal cisapride. Gastroenterology 1994;106:924–36.
16. Miedema BW, Schillie S, Simmons JW, Burgess SV, Liem T, Silver D. Small bowel motility and transit after aortic surgery. J Vasc Surg 2002;36:19–24.
17. Chapman MJ, Fraser RJ, Bryant LK, et al. Gastric emptying and the organization of antro-duodenal pressures in the critically ill. Neurogastroenterol Motil 2008; 20:27–35.
18. Toumadre JP, Barclay M, Fraser R, et al. Small intestinal motor patterns in critically ill patients after major abdominal surgery. Am J Gastroenterol 2001;96:2418–26.
19. Dive A, Miesse C, Jamart J, Evrard P, Gonzalez M, Installe E. Duodenal motor response to continuous enteral feeding is impaired in mechanically ventilated critically ill patients. Clin Nutr 1994;13:302–6.
20. Bosscha K, Nieuwenhuijs VB, Vos A, Samsom M, Roelofs JM, Akkermans LM. Gastrointestinal motility and gastric tube feeding in mechanically ventilated patients. Crit Care Med 1998;26:1510–7.
21. Dive A, Foret F, Jamart J, Bulpa P, Installe E. Effect of dopamine on gastrointestinal motility during critical illness. Intensive Care Med 2000;26:901–7.
22. Moore FA, Cocanour CS, McKinley BA, et al. Migrating motility complexes persist after severe traumatic shock in patients who tolerate enteral nutrition. J Trauma 2001;51:1075–82.

23. Fraser RJ, Ritz M, Di Matteo AC, et al. Distal small bowel motility and lipid absorption in patients following abdominal aortic aneurysm repair surgery. World J Gastroenterol 2006;12:582–7.
24. Deane AM, Summers MJ, Zaknic AV, et al. Glucose absorption and small intestinal transit in critical illness. Crit Care Med 2011.
25. Rauch S, Krueger K, Turan A, Roewer N, Sessler DI. Determining small intestinal transit time and pathomorphology in critically ill patients using video capsule technology. Intensive Care Med 2009;35:1054–9.
26. Caenepeel P, Janssens J, Vantrappen G, Eyssen H, Coremans G. Interdigestive myoelectric complex in germ-free rats. Dig Dis Sci 1989;34:1180–4.
27. Husebye E, Hellstrom PM, Midtvedt T. Intestinal microflora stimulates myoelectric activity of rat small intestine by promoting cyclic initiation and aboral propagation of migrating myoelectric complex. Dig Dis Sci 1994;39:946–56.
28. Svenberg T, Christofides ND, Fitzpatrick ML, Areola-Ortiz F, Bloom SR, Welbourn RB. Interdigestive biliary output in man: relationship to fluctuations in plasma motilin and effect of atropine. Gut 1982;23:1024–8.
29. MacFie J, Reddy BS, Gatt M, Jain PK, Sowdi R, Mitchell CJ. Bacterial translocation studied in 927 patients over 13 years. Br J Surg 2006;93:87–93.
30. Brener W, Hendrix TR, McHugh PR. Regulation of the gastric emptying of glucose. Gastroenterology 1983;85:76–82.
31. Li Y, Owyang C. Musings on the wanderer: what's new in our understanding of vago-vagal reflexes? V. Remodeling of vagus and enteric neural circuitry after vagal injury. Am J Physiol Gastrointest Liver Physiol 2003;285:G461–9.
32. Hall KE, el-Sharkawy TY, Diamant NE. Vagal control of canine postprandial upper gastrointestinal motility. Am J Physiol 1986;250(4 Pt 1):G501–10.
33. Thompson DG, Ritchie HD, Wingate DL. Patterns of small intestinal motility in duodenal ulcer patients before and after vagotomy. Gut 1982;23:517–23.
34. Liddle RA, Morita ET, Conrad CK, Williams JA. Regulation of gastric emptying in humans by cholecystokinin. J Clin Invest 1986;77:992–6.
35. Yamagishi T, Debas HT. Cholecystokinin inhibits gastric emptying by acting on both proximal stomach and pylorus. Am J Physiol 1978;234:E375–8.
36. Fraser KA, Davison JS. Meal-induced c-fos expression in brain stem is not dependent on cholecystokinin release. Am J Physiol 1993;265(1 Pt 2):R235–9.
37. Stacher G, Steinringer H, Schmierer G, Schneider C, Winklehner S. Cholecystokinin octapeptide decreases intake of solid food in man. Peptides 1982;3:133–6.
38. Borovicka J, Kreiss C, Asal K, et al. Role of cholecystokinin as a regulator of solid and liquid gastric emptying in humans. Am J Physiol 1996;271(3 Pt 1):G448–53.
39. Fried M, Erlacher U, Schwizer W, et al. Role of cholecystokinin in the regulation of gastric emptying and pancreatic enzyme secretion in humans. Studies with the cholecystokinin-receptor antagonist loxiglumide. Gastroenterology 1991;101: 503–11.
40. Rayner CK, Park HS, Doran SM, Chapman IM, Horowitz M. Effects of cholecystokinin on appetite and pyloric motility during physiological hyperglycemia. Am J Physiol Gastrointest Liver Physiol 2000;278:G98–104.
41. Nguyen N, Chapman M, Fraser R, et al. Elevated cholecystokinin levels and feed intolerance in critical illness. Crit Care Med 2006.
42. Nematy M, O'Flynn JE, Wandrag L, et al. Changes in appetite related gut hormones in intensive care unit patients: a pilot cohort study. Crit Care 2006;10:R10.
43. Nguyen NQ, Fraser RJ, Chapman M, et al. Fasting and nutrient-stimulated plasma peptide-YY levels are elevated in critical illness and associated with feed intolerance: an observational, controlled study. Crit Care 2006;10:R175.

44. Vantrappen G, Janssens J, Peeters TL, Bloom SR, Christofides ND, Hellemans J. Motilin and the interdigestive migrating motor complex in man. Dig Dis Sci 1979;24: 497–500.
45. Tomomasa T, Kuroume T, Arai H, Wakabayashi K, Itoh Z. Erythromycin induces migrating motor complex in human gastrointestinal tract. Dig Dis Sci 1986;31: 157–61.
46. Nguyen NF, Bryant R, Burgstad L, et al. Abnormalities in plasma motilin response to small intestinal nutrient stimulation in critically ill patients. Gastroenterology 2010; 138:S405.
47. Torres A, Serra-Batlles J, Ros E, et al. Pulmonary aspiration of gastric contents in patients receiving mechanical ventilation: the effect of body position. Ann Intern Med 1992;116:540–43.
48. Heyland DK, Drover JW, Dhaliwal R, Greenwood J. Optimizing the benefits and minimizing the risks of enteral nutrition in the critically ill: role of small bowel feeding. JPEN J Parenter Enteral Nutr 2002;26(6 Suppl):S51–5; discussion S56–7.
49. Ott L, Young B, Phillips R, et al. Altered gastric emptying in the head-injured patient: relationship to feeding intolerance. J Neurosurg 1991;74:738–42.
50. Chapman MJ, Besanko LK, Burgstad CM, et al. Gastric emptying of a liquid nutrient meal in the critically ill: relationship between scintigraphic and carbon breath test measurement. Gut 2011.
51. Tarling MM, Toner CC, Withington PS, Baxter MK, Whelpton R, Goldhill DR. A model of gastric emptying using paracetamol absorption in intensive care patients. Intensive Care Med 1997;23:256–60.
52. Heyland DK, Tougas G, King D, Cook DJ. Impaired gastric emptying in mechanically ventilated, critically ill patients. Intensive Care Med 1996;22:1339–44.
53. Kao CH, ChangLai SP, Chieng PU, Yen TC. Gastric emptying in head-injured patients. Am J Gastroenterol 1998;93:1108–12.
54. Spapen HD, Duinslaeger L, Diltoer M, Gillet R, Bossuyt A, Huyghens LP. Gastric emptying in critically ill patients is accelerated by adding cisapride to a standard enteral feeding protocol: results of a prospective, randomized, controlled trial. Crit Care Med 1995;23:481–5.
55. Nguyen NQ, Ng MP, Chapman M, Fraser RJ, Holloway RH. The impact of admission diagnosis on gastric emptying in critically ill patients. Crit Care 2007;11:R16.
56. McArthur CJ, Gin T, McLaren IM, Critchley JA, Oh TE. Gastric emptying following brain injury: effects of choice of sedation and intracranial pressure. Intensive Care Med 1995;21:573–6.
57. Power I, Easton JC, Todd JG, Nimmo WS. Gastric emptying after head injury. Anaesthesia 1989;44:563–6.
58. Kao CH, Ho YJ, Changlai SP, Ding HJ. Gastric emptying in spinal cord injury patients. Dig Dis Sci 1999;44:1512–5.
59. Levein NG, Thorn SE, Wattwil M. Dopamine delays gastric emptying and prolongs orocaecal transit time in volunteers. Eur J Anaesthesiol 1999;16:246–50.
60. Gati T, Gelencser F, Hideg J. The role of adrenergic receptors in the regulation of gastric motility in the rat. Z Exp Chir 1975;8:179–84.
61. Clark RA, Holdsworth CD, Rees MR, Howlett PJ. The effect on paracetamol absorption of stimulation and blockade of beta-adrenoceptors. Br J Clin Pharmacol 1980;10:555–9.
62. Nguyen NQ, Chapman MJ, Fraser RJ, et al. The effects of sedation on gastric emptying and intra-gastric meal distribution in critical illness. Intensive Care Med 2008;34:454–60.

63. Deane A, Chapman MJ, Fraser RJ, Bryant LK, Burgstad C, Nguyen NQ. Mechanisms underlying feed intolerance in the critically ill: implications for treatment. World J Gastroenterol. Aug 7 2007;13:3909–17.
64. Fraser RJ, Horowitz M, Maddox AF, Harding PE, Chatterton BE, Dent J. Hyperglycaemia slows gastric emptying in type 1 (insulin-dependent) diabetes mellitus. Diabetologia 1990;33:675–80.
65. Fraser R, Horowitz M, Dent J. Hyperglycaemia stimulates pyloric motility in normal subjects. Gut 1991;32:475–8.
66. Nguyen N, Ching K, Fraser R, Chapman M, Holloway R. The relationship between blood glucose control and intolerance to enteral feeding during critical illness. Intensive Care Med 2007;33:2085–92.
67. Lam SW, Nguyen NQ, Ching K, Chapman M, Fraser RJ, Holloway RH. Gastric feed intolerance is not increased in critically ill patients with type II diabetes mellitus. Intensive Care Med 2007;33:1740–5.
68. Nguyen NQ, Chapman M, Fraser RJ, et al. Long-standing type II diabetes mellitus is not a risk factor for slow gastric emptying in critically ill patients. Intensive Care Med 2006;32:1365–70.
69. OConnor SR, Poole J, Deane A, et al. Nasogastric feeding intolerance in the critically ill. Critical Care 2011;15(Suppl 1).
70. Zaloga GP. The myth of the gastric residual volume. Crit Care Med 2005;33:449–50.
71. Montejo JC, Minambres E, Bordeje L, et al. Gastric residual volume during enteral nutrition in ICU patients: the REGANE study. Intensive Care Med.
72. McClave SA, Lukan JK, Stefater JA, et al. Poor validity of residual volumes as a marker for risk of aspiration in critically ill patients. Crit Care Med 2005;33:324–30.
73. Chapman MJ, Fraser RJ, Matthews G, et al. Glucose absorption and gastric emptying in critical illness. Crit Care 2009;13:R140.
74. Singh G, Chaudry KI, Chudler LC, Chaudry IH. Depressed gut absorptive capacity early after trauma-hemorrhagic shock. Restoration with diltiazem treatment. Ann Surg 1991;214:712.
75. Singh G, Chaudry KI, Chudler LC, Chaudry IH. Sepsis produces early depression of gut absorptive capacity: restoration with diltiazem treatment. Am J Physiol 1992; 263(1 Pt 2):R19–23.
76. Singh G, Harkema JM, Mayberry AJ, Chaudry IH. Severe depression of gut absorptive capacity in patients following trauma or sepsis. J Trauma 1994;36:803–8; discussion 808–9.
77. Hadfield RJ, Sinclair DG, Houldsworth PE, Evans TW. Effects of enteral and parenteral nutrition on gut mucosal permeability in the critically ill. Am J Respir Crit Care Med 1995;152(5 Pt 1):1545–8.
78. Chiolero RL, Revelly JP, Berger MM, Cayeux MC, Schneiter P, Tappy L. Labeled acetate to assess intestinal absorption in critically ill patients. Crit Care Med 2003; 31:853–7.
79. Caspary WF. Physiology and pathophysiology of intestinal absorption. Am J Clin Nutr 1992;55(1 Suppl):299S–308S.
80. Hernandez G, Velasco N, Wainstein C, et al. Gut mucosal atrophy after a short enteral fasting period in critically ill patients. J Crit Care 1999;14:73–7.
81. Nguyen NQ, Burgstad C, Bellon M, et al. Delayed enteral feeding impairs intestinal carbohydrate absorption in critically ill patients. Crit Care Med 2011.
82. Drakulovic MB, Torres A, Bauer TT, Nicolas JM, Nogue S, Ferrer M. Supine body position as a risk factor for nosocomial pneumonia in mechanically ventilated patients: a randomised trial. Lancet 1999;354:1851–8.

83. Meissner W, Dohrn B, Reinhart K. Enteral naloxone reduces gastric tube reflux and frequency of pneumonia in critical care patients during opioid analgesia. Crit Care Med 2003;31:776–80.
84. Corvilain B, Abramowicz M, Fery F, et al. Effect of short-term starvation on gastric emptying in humans: relationship to oral glucose tolerance. Am J Physiol 1995;269(4 Pt 1):G512–7.
85. Nguyen NQ, Fraser RJ, Bryant LK, et al. The impact of delaying enteral feeding on gastric emptying, plasma cholecystokinin, and peptide YY concentrations in critically ill patients. Crit Care Med 2008;36:1469–74.
86. Blackshaw LA, Staunton E, Lehmann A, Dent J. Inhibition of transient LES relaxations and reflux in ferrets by GABA receptor agonists. Am J Physiol 1999;277(4 Pt 1): G867–74.
87. Lehmann A, Jensen JM, Boeckxstaens GE. GABAB receptor agonism as a novel therapeutic modality in the treatment of gastroesophageal reflux disease. Adv Pharmacol 58:287–313.
88. Jooste CA, Mustoe J, Collee G. Metoclopramide improves gastric motility in critically ill patients. Intensive Care Med 1999;25:464–8.
89. Nguyen N, Chapman, M, Fraser RJ, Bryant L, Holloway RH. Erythromycin is more effective than metoclopramide in the treatment of feed intolerance in critical illness. Crit Care Med 2006.
90. Nguyen NQ, Chapman M, Fraser RJ, Bryant LK, Burgstad C, Holloway RH. Prokinetic therapy for feed intolerance in critical illness: one drug or two? Crit Care Med 2007.
91. Nguyen NQ, Grgurinovich N, Bryant LK, et al. Plasma erythromycin concentrations predict feeding outcomes in critically ill patients with feed intolerance. Crit Care Med 39:868–71.
92. Lamian V, Rich A, Ma Zea. Characterization of agonist-induced motilin receptor trafficking and its implications for tachyphylaxis. Mol Pharmacol 2006:109–18.
93. Thielemans L, Depoortere I, Perret J, et al. Desensitization of the human motilin receptor by motilides. J Pharmacol Exp Ther 2005:1397–405.
94. Deane AM, Fraser RJ, Chapman MJ. Prokinetic drugs for feed intolerance in critical illness: current and potential therapies. Crit Care Resusc 2009;11:132–43.
95. Deane AM, Fraser RJ, Young RJ, Foreman B, O'Conner SN, Chapman MJ. Evaluation of a bedside technique for postpyloric placement of feeding catheters. Crit Care Resusc 2009;11:180–3.
96. Holzinger U, Brunner R, Miehsler W, et al. Jejunal tube placement in critically ill patients: A prospective, randomized trial comparing the endoscopic technique with the electromagnetically visualized method. Crit Care Med 39:73–7.
97. Ho KM, Dobb GJ, Webb SA. A comparison of early gastric and post-pyloric feeding in critically ill patients: a meta-analysis. Intensive Care Med 2006;32:639–49.
98. White H, Sosnowski K, Tran K, Reeves A, Jones M. A randomised controlled comparison of early post-pyloric versus early gastric feeding to meet nutritional targets in ventilated intensive care patients. Crit Care 2009;13:R187.
99. Chapman MD, et al. Glucose absorption following gastric and small intestinal nutrient administration in the critically ill. Crit Care 2011;15(Suppl).

Motility Disorders in the Patient with Neurologic Disease

Eamonn M.M. Quigley, MD, FRCP, FRCPI[a,*],
Seamus O'Mahony, MD, FRCP[b], Zaid Heetun, MB, MRCPI[a]

KEYWORDS

- Dysphagia • Gastroparesis • Pseudoobstruction
- Megacolon • Cerebrovascular disease • Parkinson disease
- Multiple sclerosis • Motor neuron disease • Myopathy
- Neurologic • Motility

As populations age, the prevalence of neurologic disease in the community continues to increase, and consultations relating to gastrointestinal motility problems in the patient afflicted with a neurologic disorder become ever more common.

Although in theory several gastrointestinal functions could be disturbed in neurologic disorders in relation either to a given disease process or to its therapy, this article focuses on the gastrointestinal function that has received the greatest attention in this context, namely, gastrointestinal motility.

GUT MOTOR FUNCTION AND ITS RELEVANCE TO NEUROLOGIC DISEASE

Given its essential role in digestion, absorption, secretion, and excretion, the gastrointestinal tract and its associated organs play an essential role in homeostasis. The various physiologic processes of the gastrointestinal tract serve these functions; thus, motility propels food, chyme, and stool and promotes mixing to increase contact time and thereby digestion. Gut muscle and nerve are integrated into a "mini-brain" and are adapted to subserve these homeostatic functions. Throughout most of the gastrointestinal tract, gut smooth muscle is arranged in two layers, an outer longitudinal layer and an inner circular layer. However, at the beginning and end of the gut, striated muscle is found in the oropharynx, upper esophageal sphincter (UES), proximal part of the esophagus, external anal sphincter, and pelvic floor muscles. In these locations, somatic innervation plays a crucial role in the regulation of swallowing and defecation; these functions are, not surprisingly, particularly prone

The authors have nothing to disclose.
[a] Department of Medicine, Alimentary Pharmabiotic Centre, University College Cork, Cork, Ireland
[b] Gastroenterology, Cork University Hospital, Cork, Ireland
* Corresponding author.
E-mail address: e.quigley@ucc.ie

Gastroenterol Clin N Am 40 (2011) 741–764
doi:10.1016/j.gtc.2011.09.008
0889-8553/11/$ – see front matter

to disruption, and in neurologic disease and dysphagia, constipation and fecal incontinence are prominent issues.

Throughout the remainder of the gut, several levels of control are evident. Myogenic regulation of motility refers to intrinsic properties of gut muscle cells and their interactions with one another. The biochemistry and molecular biology of enteric smooth muscle has much in common with its striated counterpart, thus explaining the high frequency of gut involvement in muscular dystrophies.

The next layer of control is provided by the enteric nervous system (ENS), which is now recognized as a distinct and independent division of the autonomic nervous system.[1] The ENS may represent the most important level of neuronal control of motility. It is capable of generating and modulating many functions within the gastrointestinal tract without input from the more traditional divisions of the autonomic system and central nervous system (CNS). Through variations in neuronal morphology and in the electrophysiologic properties of individual neurons, as well as through the presence of a wide variety of neurotransmitters and neuromodulatory peptides, the ENS demonstrates striking plasticity. Of relevance to any discussion of the gut in CNS disorders, it is now recognized that the ENS and CNS share many similarities, both morphologic and functional. Thus the basic organization of the ENS (neurons, ganglia, glia, an ENS-blood barrier), as well as the ultrastructure of its components, are similar to that of the CNS, and almost all neurotransmitters identified within the CNS are also found in enteric neurons. The concept of ENS involvement in neurologic disease should not, therefore, come as a great surprise.

Although the ENS is primarily responsible for the generation and modulation of most motor activities within the gut, input from autonomic nerves and the CNS also modulates motor activity. Autonomic input is now recognized to be exerted primarily though the modulation of ENS activity rather than through a direct input to effector cells in the gut, be they smooth muscle or epithelial secretory cells. Given the prevalence of autonomic dysfunction in a number of neurologic syndromes, as well as the existence of a number of primary and secondary disorders of autonomic function, disturbed autonomic modulation of gut motor function may be an important contributory factor to symptomatology in some scenarios.

It is now evident that the gut has important sensory functions. Although usually subconscious, gut sensation may be relayed to and perceived within the CNS. Sensory input is also fundamental to several reflex events in the gut, such as the viscerovisceral reflexes that coordinate function along the gut.[2] The role of sensory dysfunction in the mediation of common symptoms, such as abdominal pain and nausea, in the patient with CNS disease with gastrointestinal manifestations has not been extensively investigated, however.

THE PATHOGENESIS OF GASTROINTESTINAL DYSFUNCTION IN NEUROLOGIC DISEASE

Whereas a whole range of disease processes affecting central, peripheral, and autonomic nervous systems may affect gut motor function, the two predominant neurologic disorders encountered in gastrointestinal practice are cerebrovascular disease and parkinsonism.

Cerebrovascular Disease

Because of the aforementioned location of the swallowing center in the brain stem, it should come as no surprise that severe dysphagia can occur as a result of brainstem infarcts, especially if bilateral. Dysphagia following cortical strokes is a well-recognized and common complication, occurring in up to 50% of ischemic strokes,[3,4] and its occurrence is associated with increased mortality and impaired functional outcome. Poststroke dysphagia is multifactorial and is largely attributable to oropharyngeal dysfunction. Abnormalities include incomplete lip closure, poor tongue movement, increased pooling, weak laryngeal elevation, and an increased frequency of airway penetration.[5] Elegant imaging studies have provided considerable insights into the pathophysiology of dysphagia and its recovery in hemispheric strokes.[4–8] These studies have emphasized the importance of cortical as well as brain stem control in the regulation of the swallowing mechanism.[8] In humans, one hemisphere usually demonstrates dominance in the control of swallowing.[4,5,8] At the cortical level, ischemic events that involve projections from the precentral gyrus to the internal capsule are most likely to be complicated by dysphagia.[9] Brain stem strokes are especially likely to result in dysphagia, which may be slower to recover from and is more likely to result in aspiration. Given the role of the dorsal motor nucleus of the vagus in the medulla in the control of the smooth muscle esophagus and lower esophageal function, peristaltic dysfunction and gastroesophageal reflux would be expected in the stroke patient; however, there have been few studies of these aspects of esophageal function in the aftermath of acute stroke.[9,10]

The good news is that, thanks to neuronal plasticity within the CNS,[4,5,7] dysphagia resolves spontaneously in most cortical stroke patients within 2 weeks of the ischemic insult.[4] Recovery seems to represent assumption by the unaffected hemisphere of the cortical control of swallowing rather than recovery of function in the damaged area; swallowing improvement may therefore occur independent of any recovery of limb function. This aspect of recovery is important and suggests that one should not be rushed into interventions in the interim but rather maintain close observation for risks for and the occurrence of aspiration.[11]

Although little studied, there is indirect evidence to suggest that gastric emptying may be delayed following an acute stroke,[9] which may have implications for feeding and drug administration. Stroke is also associated with constipation and anorectal dysfunction[12] including incontinence, and instances of intestinal pseudo-obstruction have been reported.[9] In contrast to swallowing function, gastric, small intestinal, colonic, and anorectal motor or sensory function have been little studied in the context of stroke, and therefore the pathophysiology of complications involving these parts of the gastrointestinal tract is less clearly understood. Whereas immobility may play some role, it is likely that cortical regulation of colonic and anorectal physiology is more important.

Parkinson Disease

Idiopathic Parkinson disease (PD) causes widespread and sometimes severe derangement of gastrointestinal motility.[13–16] There are two basic contributors to gastrointestinal dysfunction in PD. First, striatal muscle dysfunction in the oropharynx, proximal esophagus, and anal canal is based on the same neurologic abnormalities that cause the cardinal manifestations of this disorder. The second component, dysfunction in the smooth muscle parts of the gastrointestinal tract, is less well understood but may reflect pathology in the autonomic and/or ENS systems.[17–20] Indeed, neuropathologic changes reminiscent of CNS Parkinson features, such as dopamine depletion[19] and the presence of Lewy neuritis,[20] have been demonstrated in the myenteric and submucosal plexuses.

The pathogenesis of dysphagia in PD was studied in detail by Ali and colleagues[21] in a detailed videofluoromanometric study of the swallowing process. The most prominent abnormalities, disturbed tongue movement and reduced amplitude of pharyngeal peristalsis, conspired to impair upper sphincter opening and thereby retard bolus passage into the esophagus. Cricopharyngeal bars and hypopharyngeal diverticula have also been described in PD.[22] Involvement of the dorsal motor nucleus of the vagus and of central noradrenergic neurons, as well as the ENS of the esophagus, may contribute to the occurrence of esophageal dysphagia in PD.[17,23]

With regard to the stomach, small intestine, and colon, similar hypotheses have been advanced to explain the high prevalence of symptoms related to these organs in PD,[24] but in these regions the role of autonomic and ENS pathologic abnormalities looms large. The contribution of autonomic dysfunction is illustrated by the higher prevalence of gastrointestinal symptoms as well as postural instability among patients with a PD variant, multiple system atrophy, in which autonomic dysfunction is especially common.[25] For some of these symptoms, such as nausea, the contribution of antiparkinsonian medications and dopaminergics in particular must be remembered.

Delayed gastric emptying has been well-documented in PD,[26–30] and delayed emptying of solids has been linked in some studies to the severity of motor impairment.[28,30] Here again, the impact of levodopa must be accounted for.[27] The association between gastric emptying delay and the presence of levodopa response fluctuations,[26] coupled with irregular patterns of drug absorption[31] and the documentation of improved symptom control with intrajejunal[32] or transdermal[33] administration of antiparkinsonian drugs, underlines the potential clinical relevance of gastric emptying delay: by retarding drug delivery and absorption, gastroparesis could induce or further exacerbate response fluctuations. Several factors, however, limit the interpretation of reports of delayed gastric emptying and its association with upper gastrointestinal symptoms in PD. These factors include variations in patient population studied (eg, age, gender, disease severity, study location), the definition of gastroparesis, and the methodology used to assess gastric emptying rate (meal, test technique, study protocol, and manner of interpretation). Variations between studies in these parameters make it difficult to attempt real comparisons or draw firm conclusions. Nevertheless, delayed gastric emptying may occur in as many as 70% to 100% of PD patients attending specialist neurology clinics; the prevalence of symptomatic gastroparesis in PD, however, remains unknown. Indeed, there has been a lack of a consistent correlation between gastric emptying rate and upper gastrointestinal symptoms in PD. Although it is reasonable to assume that gastroparesis contributes to the weight loss that has been well-documented in PD,[34] it is unclear whether nutrient delivery is affected by delayed gastric emptying, and a relationship between delayed gastric emptying and weight loss is yet to be demonstrated. Electrogastrography has also been used to study gastric motor activity in PD, but correlations with symptoms have been poor.[35,36] Parenthetically, *Helicobacter pylori* and *Helicobacter heilmannii* infection have been implicated not only in contributing to gastrointestinal symptoms and weight loss in PD,[37] but also in systemic proinflammatory cytokine activation[37] and even in the pathogenesis of PD itself.[38,39]

Orocecal and colonic transit times are significantly prolonged in patients with PD,[40–43] and small intestinal bacterial overgrowth, presumed to be consequent to impaired small intestinal motility, has been documented.[44]

Constipation, a common and at times dominant symptom in PD,[13–16,24] is probably multifactorial, with delayed colonic transit, anorectal dysfunction,[41,43] drug therapy, and reduced physical activity all contributing to the problem. Difficulty with the act of defecation may be an especially distressing symptom for affected patients; this symptom seems to be associated with PD severity, and its pathophysiology is based on the involvement of the anal sphincter and pelvic floor musculature by the PD process[41,45–47] (**Fig. 1**). Accordingly, responses have been documented for apomorphine injection.[48]

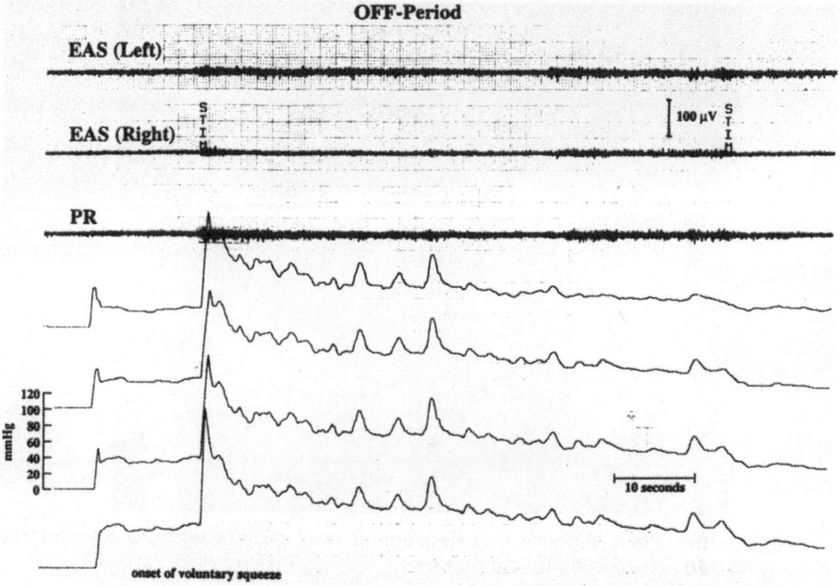

Fig. 1. Abnormal anal sphincter squeeze effort in PD. Simultaneous electromyography (recording from external anal sphincter [EAS] and puborectalis [PR]) and manometry (multilumen catheter assembly straddling the anal sphincter) demonstrating response to voluntary squeeze. Note rapidly decaying squeeze response with superimposed phasic pressure fluctuations.

Megacolon, at times requiring surgical intervention and even resulting in perforation and fatal outcome, has been well-documented in PD (**Fig. 2**).

Motor Neuron Disease (Amyotrophic Lateral Sclerosis)

Motor neuron disease (amyotrophic lateral sclerosis, or ALS) features the progressive degeneration of motor neurons in the brain, brainstem, and spinal cord. When, as often happens, the cranial nerve nuclei become involved, swallowing is disrupted and difficulties ensue, and severe and potentially fatal aspiration-related events can occur. Unfortunately, the natural history is typically one of inexorable progression, and issues regarding alternative routes of feeding and fluid administration inevitably arise. Colonic function is also affected, and delayed transit in the right and left colon have been described[49]; it has been suggested that involvement of the autonomic nervous system might explain these findings.[49,50] Fortunately, the pelvic floor muscles and Onuf nucleus motor neurons are relatively spared in ALS and, although involvement of the external anal sphincter has been documented by some[51] but not others,[52] fecal incontinence is infrequent.[51]

Multiple Sclerosis

Among patients with long-standing (>10 years' duration) multiple sclerosis (MS) in Finland, mortality rates from pneumonia and gastrointestinal disorders were four-fold more common than in the general population.[53]

Dysphagia, previously thought to be rare, has in more recent studies been reported in up to 30% to 40% of MS patients and, although all phases of swallowing can be

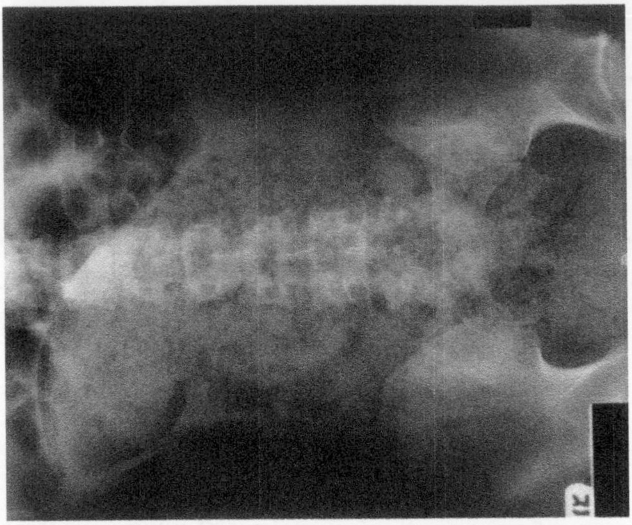

Fig. 2. Megarectum. Plain abdominal radiograph from a patient with PD demonstrating enormously dilated rectum full of fecal material.

impaired, oropharyngeal dysphagia is the most common manifestation, and abnormalities in pharyngeal and cricopharyngeal function have been described.[54,55] Dysphagia prevalence correlates with disease duration and extent[54]; it is reasonable to assume that aspiration may be a significant contributor to the previously mentioned excess deaths from pneumonia. When studied, dysphagia has, not surprisingly, been linked to evidence of brainstem involvement.[55]

Delayed gastric emptying,[56] isolated cases of gastroparesis,[57–60] and even one instance of gastric perforation[61] have been reported in MS, and their cause has been attributed to autonomic dysfunction of central origin.[62] In one small series, parallel improvements in neurologic and gastric emptying function were documented in response to corticosteroid therapy.[60]

In patients with MS, constipation is reported among 29% to 43% and fecal incontinence in over 50%, and these conditions exert a deleterious impact on quality of life.[63,64] Bowel involvement is less common than bladder involvement and its pathophysiology less well-understood.[65] Incontinence in MS has been attributed to abnormal rectosigmoid compliance and rectoanal reflexes, reduced rectal sensation, and loss of voluntary control of the external anal sphincter musculature,[66] and constipation has been attributed to slow colon transit and paradoxical contraction of the puborectalis muscle.[67,68]

Autonomic and Peripheral Neuropathies

Given its ever-increasing worldwide prevalence, diabetic autonomic neuropathy is by far the most common autonomic neuropathy encountered in clinical practice. However, involvement of other pathologic processes, especially those involving the ENS[69] and the interstitial cells of Cajal, must be noted.[70] Gastrointestinal involvement in diabetes can affect any or all parts of the gastrointestinal tract with delayed esophageal transit, gastroparesis, intestinal pseudo-obstruction, constipation, and incontinence being well-documented, and delayed gastric emptying reported in 30%

to 50% of outpatients with longstanding type 1 or type 2 diabetes.[71] Hyperglycemia delays gastric emptying in normal subjects and in diabetes; for patients with diabetes, this phenomenon must be accounted for in the performance and interpretation of gastric emptying studies and considered in patient management.

Gastrointestinal involvement occurs to a variable extent in the many types of autonomic peripheral neuropathies.[72] Upper gastrointestinal symptoms (early satiety, nausea, and vomiting) as well as constipation are common in autoimmune autonomic neuropathies.[73] Paralytic ileus is a common feature of the rare acute autonomic and sensory neuropathy.[74]

Bulbar and oculomotor nerves are less commonly affected in the most common form of Guillain-Barré syndrome (GBS) seen in Europe and North America (approximately 85% of cases), which is the sensory-motor form referred to as acute inflammatory demyelinating polyradiculoneuropathy. However, bulbar and oculomotor nerve involvement is a common feature of other, less common, subtypes such as Miller Fisher syndrome.[75,76] Bulbar involvement can lead to oropharyngeal dysphagia and respiratory difficulties. Autonomic dysfunction is commonly detectable in GBS but is usually of minor clinical importance.[75] Delayed gastric emptying, gastroparesis, constipation, diarrhea, and fecal incontinence have all been described in GBS.[77] The gastrointestinal tract has a role in the pathogenesis of GBS; 15% to 40% of cases of GBS in the west have followed infection with *Campylobacter jejuni*.[78]

Muscle Disease

Myopathy and muscular dystrophy

Nasal aspiration is a prominent feature of myopathic involvement of the oropharyngeal musculature. Weakness of the tongue and pharyngeal and laryngeal musculature may result in ineffective bolus transfer, retention of components of the bolus in the valleculae or hypopharynx, and/or aspiration. Whereas a large number of myopathic disorders may involve the swallowing mechanism, oropharyngeal dysphagia is a characteristic feature of oculopharyngeal dystrophy.[79] This form of muscular dystrophy features an autosomal dominant inheritance and presents with ptosis, oropharyngeal dysphagia, and proximal limb weakness.[80] Whereas gastrointestinal involvement has been described in a number of muscular dystrophies,[81–84] it has been most extensively documented in myotonic dystrophy and Duchenne muscular dystrophy. Gastrointestinal symptoms in myotonic dystrophy include dysphagia, aspiration, early satiety, nausea, vomiting, epigastric pain, constipation, difficult defecation, abdominal pain, pseudo-obstruction, and fecal incontinence.[85] Of these, abdominal pain, dysphagia, vomiting, diarrhea, coughing while eating, and fecal incontinence were the most common in one survey[86]; up to 25% of patients consider gastrointestinal involvement as the most disabling feature of their disease.[87] Functional correlates include impaired upper and lower esophageal sphincter pressures, esophageal peristalsis, and even aperistalsis[88] leading to esophageal dilation[85]; delayed gastric emptying and gastroparesis[89–91]; abnormal small intestinal motility[92,93] leading to pseudo-obstruction[94,95]; and impaired anal sphincter function.[96,97] Gastric volvulus[98] and megacolon[99] have been described. In Duchenne dystrophy, esophageal symptoms such as dysphagia and aspiration are not common,[100,101] although esophageal manometric abnormalities have been described.[102] In contrast, gastric motor dysfunction is an early feature,[103] resulting in hypomotility and gastroparesis,[104] which can be profound and result in acute gastroparesis and gastric dilatation.[105,106] Although when measured, orocecal transit time was found to be normal,[107] instances of intestinal pseudo-obstruction have been reported.[108]

Myasthenia gravis

Because the muscles controlled by the cranial nerves are commonly involved in myasthenia, dysphagia is prevalent.[109] Severity of dysphagia is variable, ranging from fatigable swallowing difficulty evident only after a considerable duration of effort to constant difficulty, a poor prognostic sign. Two cases of intestinal obstruction have been described as a paraneoplastic manifestation of thymomas associated with myasthenia.[110]

Alzheimer disease and other dementias

Pilot data indicate that swallowing duration is significantly delayed in Alzheimer disease, the delay being located principally at the pharyngeal level.[111] There are no published data on the influence of Alzheimer disease and other dementias on gastric or small intestinal motility. Constipation is a well-described and common problem among patients with dementia.[112] Despite this fact, there are no published studies of gastrointestinal motility in dementia. One large-scale retrospective survey of the medical records of 4 million patients discharged from United States veterans hospitals has shown that Alzheimer disease was associated with significantly increased risk of constipation, megacolon, volvulus, and intestinal impaction compared with patients without neurologic or psychiatric disease.[113]

ISSUES IN CLINICAL PRACTICE

Assessment

Oropharyngeal dysphagia

The evaluation of oropharyngeal dysphagia is firmly based on two modalities: the bedside clinical assessment and dynamic imaging of the swallowing mechanism, both preferably performed in collaboration with a speech and language therapist with expertise in the assessment and management of dysphagia. The imaging modality most commonly used and most extensively documented in the literature is videofluoroscopy, which, when performed by an experienced clinician, can evaluate the various components of the oropharyngeal phase of the swallow, define dysfunction, and predict therapeutic response. For example, the observation of impaired laryngeal closure predicts tracheal, and soft palate dysfunction, nasopharyngeal aspiration. Impaired UES opening leads to dysphagia, postswallow aspiration, and, in the case of cricopharyngeal bars, diverticulum formation. Tongue dysfunction with attendant impaired bolus propulsion leads to a sluggish, misdirected bolus. Finally, an impaired pharyngeal contraction results in postswallow residue in the valleculae and pyriform sinuses with the risk of postswallow aspiration.[114] A key issue for the clinician is the detection of aspiration and/or the determination of risk for aspiration. Unfortunately, such traditional clinical signs as the gag reflex have not stood the test of time. Even when performed by a skilled evaluator and according to a standard and detailed protocol, the bedside assessment of swallowing has its limitations. In one prospective study among patients with acute stroke, sensitivity was only 47%, whereas specificity was 86% for the presence of aspiration.[115] Among the various symptoms and signs evaluated, a weak voluntary cough and the presence of any alteration in conscious level were the most predictive, the combination having a sensitivity of 75% and specificity of 91%.[115] Furthermore, a prior study from the same group found that the routine use of videofluoroscopy added little to the bedside assessment in the detection of aspiration.[116] Indeed, it has been pointed out repeatedly that videofluoroscopy was never designed as a test for aspiration. The bottom line: current commonly used methods for the prediction of aspiration have their limitations and should be interpreted with caution. It is evident, however, that clinical and radiologic evaluation by a multidisciplinary team continues to be the best approach.

The esophageal phase of swallowing is primarily a function of the smooth muscle esophagus and is regulated centrally via vagal afferents and peripherally by the intrinsic properties of esophageal smooth muscle. The assessment of the esophageal phase of swallowing is dealt with in detail by Dr Kahrilas elsewhere in this issue.

Gastroparesis

Modalities used to diagnose gastroparesis include scintigraphy (still the gold standard) where the time taken to empty a solid radiolabeled test meal is measured. Optimum results are obtained if scintigraphy is performed according to a standardized protocol and scanning is extended to at least 4 hours postprandially.[117] Regional gastric emptying can be used to assess fundic and antral function. Dual-labeled scintigraphy can offer insights into the differential handling by the stomach of liquids and solids. Based on its ability to identify transit into the duodenum by a sudden and profound change in pH, the wireless motility capsule is able to estimate the rate of gastric emptying and provide estimates of gastric and colonic motor function in the absence of radiation exposure, although availability remains limited and the costprohibitive for many.[118] Other modalities under evaluation for use in the diagnosis and research of gastroparesis include the octanoic acid breath test, functional magnetic resonance imaging (MRI), and both 2-dimensional and 3-dimensional ultrasonography.[119]

Chronic intestinal pseudo-obstruction

Although chronic intestinal pseudo-obstruction (CIP) may involve any part of the gastrointestinal tract and may result in symptoms related to that organ (eg, gastroesophageal reflux disease, dysphagia, achalasia, gastroparesis, constipation, megacolon), symptoms referable to small intestinal obstruction classically dominate the clinical picture. The typical history of the patient with CIP is repeated admissions with symptoms, signs, and radiologic evidence of "obstruction" with no convincing cause for obstruction being found. Unfortunately, these patients have usually been subjected to a number of fruitless laparotomies before the diagnosis is even entertained. Attention to the clinical context should prompt suspicion of CIP. CIP has been described in association with diabetic neuropathy, myotonic dystrophy, dermatomyositis, and amyloidosis, and iatrogenic cases have complicated therapy with antiparkinsonian medications, phenothiazines, and tricyclic antidepressants. Details of the clinical features, diagnostic approach to, and management of CIP are provided by Dr De Giorgio and colleagues elsewhere in this issue.

Colonic inertia and megacolon

Colonic motor dysfunction is common in neurologic disorders and may manifest as slow transit constipation or acute or chronic megacolon.

Acute megacolon. Acute colonic pseudo-obstruction, or Ogilvie syndrome, is defined as an acute dilatation of the colon without evidence of mechanical obstruction distal to the dilated segment.[120] Progressive abdominal distention is the clinical hallmark of this condition. Lower abdominal pain is present in 60% to 80% of patients, and nausea and vomiting is present in 50%. It is important to realize that although the vast majority of patients with Ogilvie syndrome are completely constipated, megacolon can develop in individuals who continue to pass both stool and flatus. Only 40% of patients will have hypoactive or absent bowel sounds. The overall risk of perforation in Ogilvie syndrome is low, in the region of 3%, but mortality following perforation in this context may be as high as 50%. Cecal diameter is valuable in predicting risk of perforation; a diameter in excess of 9 cm is abnormal, and when greater than 12 cm indicates a significant risk of perforation.

Chronic megacolon. Chronic megacolon has been described in PD, MS, motor neuron disease, Alzheimer disease, and autonomic neuropathies and in relation to spinal cord injury, among others. In many instances chronic megacolon may be asymptomatic and discovered only on clinical or radiologic examination; depending on the level of consciousness and cognitive function, the patient may be aware of abdominal distension and discomfort. Although the risk of perforation with chronic megacolon is apparently low, instances have been reported in association with neurologic disease, and fatal outcomes have occurred.

Constipation. Two related aspects of colonic function are amenable to clinical testing: transit and contractile activity. Of these two, colon transit is by far the most widely used, and its popularity owes much to the validation of a simple test of transit: the radioopaque marker study. Using ingested radioopaque markers and following their movement through the colon by timed abdominal radiographs, an accurate and reproducible assessment of overall colonic transit can be obtained. More accurate and dynamic assessments of colon transit, including the determination of transit within segments of various segments of the colon, can be obtained from radioisotopic approaches, although these methodologies have been largely confined to a few centers and to clinical research protocols.[121] Smart Pill technology has also been used to measure colon transit and in an initial study in constipation, a good correlation was noted between transit measurements obtained by this technique and the traditional radioopaque marker method.[118]

In contrast to these relatively simple techniques, colonic manometry presents formidable challenges, foremost being positioning the catheter assembly in the first place and ensuring that it retains its position throughout the period of study. Furthermore, patterns of colonic motility are poorly defined and subject to tremendous variation between normal individuals, not to mention in disease states. The American Neurogastroenterology and Motility Society consensus statement on intraluminal measurement of colonic motility concluded that "in children with chronic constipation, colonic phasic pressure measurements can identify patterns suggestive of neuropathy and predict success of antegrade enemas via cecostomy."[122] The society's stand regarding colonic manometry in adults was more circumspect; it stated that manometry "may be used to document severe motor dysfunction (colonic inertia) prior to colectomy." There are no data on the utility of this approach in the patient with neurologic disease.

Anorectal sphincter and pelvic floor dysfunction

Two clinical problems that may coexist may be addressed in the assessment of anorectal and pelvic floor muscle function: fecal incontinence and difficult defecation (anismus, pelvic floor dyssynergia). Digital rectal examination, performed by a skilled clinician, has been shown to be of value[123] and, in the appropriate clinical context, endoscopic and/or radiologic studies may be required to uncover other abnormalities such as inflammatory bowel disease or a rectal neoplasm. In the evaluation of the patient with fecal incontinence, both endoanal ultrasound and endoanal MRI are widely used to define anatomic (usually obstetric or postsurgical) defects in the internal and external anal sphincters, with ultrasound being the preferred modality for the former and MRI for the latter.[124] Static images of the anorectal angle can be obtained during defecography (whether performed using fluoroscopy or MRI), which can also follow the transit of feces (or, more usually, a simulated stool) through the rectum and anal canal using standard contrast imaging, scintigraphy, or MRI. The first two modalities involve radiation exposure and the use of a customized "throne" on which the patient sits and performs various maneuvers following the insertion of a material to simulate the consistency of feces into the rectum. In this manner the behavior of the pelvic floor musculature can be recorded as the patient attempts to retain or expel stool. MRI offers many advantages over barium defecography but for a truly physiologic test requires a dedicated "open" system, a facility that is available at only a few highly specialized centers.[124] Anorectal manometry has been used for decades to assess the integrity of the internal and external sphincters and is a well-established technique for the identification of Hirschsprung disease and the definition of poor sphincter tone in patients with incontinence. In the latter context, the clinician can go on to use manometry as the basis for biofeedback approaches to improving sphincter function. A variety of manometric assemblies have been used: multiple balloon, perfused catheter, solid-state, and high-resolution. In the most commonly used approach, a perfused catheter assembly incorporating multiple radially arrayed (to allow for sphincter asymmetry) closely-spaced side holes (typically 0.5 to 1 cm apart) with an inflatable balloon at its tip is placed in the rectum and anal canal so that the sensors straddle the sphincter, previously identified by a series of slow pull-through maneuvers. Most recently the technique of high-resolution manometry, now widely used in studies of the esophagus, has been used in the anorectum and has been shown to correlate well with conventional water perfused manometry yet provide greater anatomic detail.[125]

Management

Oropharyngeal dysphagia

In cases of less severe impairment in which aspiration is not an issue and the patient is willing and able to cooperate, a number of maneuvers combined with dietary changes can be taught to compensate for impaired laryngeal (chin tuck and "supraglottic swallow") or nasopharyngeal closure, UES opening (Mendelsohn maneuver, which helps to raise the larynx and facilitate UES opening), and impaired pharyngeal clearance.[126,127]

There have been isolated reports of cricopharyngeal myotomy and botulinum toxin injection into the cricopharyngeus in patients with PD[22] and MS,[55] respectively, who seemed to have oropharyngeal dysphagia related to holdup at the cricopharyngues muscle. Given the predilection of such patients to aspiration, these are not approaches to embarked upon lightly.

As for the assessment of oropharyngeal dysphagia in the neurologic patient, management must be guided by a team approach, being mindful of the severity of the dysphagia, nutritional status of the patient, nature of the underlying illness, general health status, and above all of the wishes and well-being of the patient.[128,129]

To PEG or not to PEG

Despite initial enthusiasm for the insertion of percutaneous endoscopic gastrostomy (PEG) tubes in patients with Alzheimer disease and other dementias, it is now clear that PEG does not prolong life or relieve suffering for these patients but is accompanied by significant risk, including local infection and aspiration. Less than 40% of older patients in whom a PEG tube is placed survive beyond 1 year after the procedure, and survival was even lower among those with malignancy or advanced age.[130] Furthermore, the likelihood of aspiration may be enhanced and not, as commonly believed, prevented by PEG feeding.[131] Nevertheless, gastroenterologists continue to come under pressure from families and nursing homes.[132,133] (In some instances these patients will not be accepted without a PEG tube in situ.) It is also evident that the caloric requirements of these patients may have been overestimated and that oral feeding, despite its difficulty, may not only be adequate but more appropriate in many instances.[134,135] It should come as no surprise, therefore, that a recent Cochrane systematic review concluded that there was "insufficient evidence to suggest that enteral tube feeding (including by PEG) was beneficial in patients with advanced dementia."[136]

As already mentioned, dysphagia is common in acute stroke but is often transient and, if persistent, a predictor of a poor prognosis in terms of survival and neurologic recovery. Here again, the role of PEG feeding has undergone a significant reappraisal with the publication of the FOOD trial, which showed that early PEG feeding (as compared with nasogastric tube feeding) was associated with an increased risk of death or poor outcome.[137]

In considering PEG placement in patients with oropharyngeal dysphagia related to chronic neurologic diseases such as MS or ALS and where dysphagia is of such severity as to make oral intake impossible and/or where aspiration is a real threat, a number of factors must be considered. If aspiration is deemed significant and especially if recovery is unlikely or progression inevitable, alternative routes of nutrition must be considered if ethically justified. It must be emphasized that PEG placement offers no significant protection against aspiration pneumonia[138]; indeed, aspiration pneumonia is the most common cause of death in PEG-fed patients. A number of factors contribute including the aspiration of colonized oral secretions and/or gastric contents.[139] The latter will, of course, be aggravated by the presence of gastroparesis. If aspiration is not a significant risk but alternative routes of nutrition are required, PEG placement should be considered, bearing in mind the very particular clinical context that presents itself to the gastroenterologist. A systematic review by the American Academy of Neurology concluded that although enteral feeding via a PEG tube "probably" prolonged survival in ALS, there was no evidence regarding PEG impact on quality of life, and there were insufficient data to support or refute specific timing of PEG insertion.[140] The organization did suggest that an ALS patient would be exposed to less risk if a PEG tube was placed while forced vital capacity was above 50% of predicted.[140] Gastrostomy tubes may also be placed radiologically (radiologically guided gastrostomy; RIG) A comparative study among ALS patients could detect no differences in terms of complications or survival. RIG may be more feasible and safe than PEG among ALS patients with significant ventilatory compromise, however.[141]

Gastroparesis

In the patient with symptomatic gastroparesis, dehydration and electrolyte abnormalities should be corrected by oral or intravenous routes, as appropriate. Gastric decompression by nasogastric suction remains an important component of management in the acute stage. Malnutrition develops in many patients who have chronic established gastroparesis as a result of inadequate oral intake and vomiting. Therefore, attention to diet[142,143] and nutrition remains of paramount importance. Low roughage low-fat diets are recommended. When oral intake fails, jejunostomy feeding may be considered. Percutaneous or, preferably, surgical placement of a combined gastrostomy-jejunostomy tube simultaneously decompresses the stomach and permits enteral nutrition.[144]

Gastroparesis may be complicated by the development of phytobezoars. When symptomatic, these may be approached endoscopically or surgically, but enzyme dissolution and Coca-Cola lavage are less invasive alternatives. By infusing Coca-Cola in a volume of 3 L over 12 hours, in one study complete resolution of all 5 cases of bezoar was recorded.[145]

Although the real clinical impact of chronic hyperglycemia on motility is unclear, it seems reasonable to advise that diabetic control should be optimized in patients with diabetic gastroenteropathy. In diabetes, interactions between blood sugar level and gastric emptying rate are critical to nutrient delivery, and thus to postprandial glycemic control.

Few effective pharmacologic agents remain available to the clinician for the management of gastroparesis.[146] Although many new agents have been evaluated, few have proven either sufficiently effective or adequately safe to merit approval for human use. Progress in this area has also been hampered by our poor understanding of the basic pathophysiology of these disorders.[147]

In terms of pharmacologic therapy, metoclopramide or domperidone (where available), and erythromycin have the best evidence for efficacy in gastroparesis. Whereas erythromycin should probably be reserved for intravenous use in the acutely ill patient, metoclopramide remains the sole option for long-term oral therapy in the United States. This agent also has significant side effect issues, of which the prescribing clinician must be fully apprised.

Nausea may be a significant problem for many of these patients and may respond to concomitant administration of an antiemetic. In these circumstances, an antiemetic such as a phenothiazine derivative or a 5-HT_3 antagonist should be used and can often be used successfully as circumstances may require. In choosing a particular antiemetic, attention should be paid to the appropriateness of available formulations, duration of action, and cost.

Given the paucity of pharmacologic options, other approaches have been explored for the patient with intractable and disabling gastroparesis. The perendoscopic injection of botulinum toxin into the pyloric muscle ring has been shown to be effective, albeit in the short term, in the symptomatic relief of gastroparesis, in accelerating gastric emptying, and in suppressing isolated pyloric pressure waves.[148–152]

In 1997, gastric stimulation was proposed as an alternative for individuals with intractable gastroparesis.[153,154] Although results in uncontrolled trials have been promising in terms of symptom relief,[153–155] nutritional status,[156] diabetic control,[157] and pancreatic function,[158] the results of the only double-blind controlled trial to date were less impressive.[159,160] Other studies have shown little impact on long-term outcome,[161] and this procedure is not without complications.[159,162] The precise mode of action of gastric stimulation remains uncertain and may be independent of an acceleration of gastric emptying.

In a small number of patients, usually those with long-standing, complicated type 1 diabetes, severely symptomatic and apparently intractable gastroparesis develops. Near-total gastrectomy with Roux-en-Y anastomosis has been performed for such patients, and good results have been reported, albeit in small series.[163–165] Furthermore, although results in terms of gastric function may be good, many of these patients go on to develop renal failure and other complications of diabetes.[164]

For the patient with PD and gastric emptying delay, it is critical to avoid metoclopramide in view of its central antidopaminergic effects; domperidone and mosapride, where available, may provide some potential therapeutic solutions. The main aim of pharmacologic therapy in correcting delayed gastric emptying in PD is primarily to reduce response fluctuations rather than deal with upper gastrointestinal symptoms. If pharmacologic approaches do not work, jejunal[32] or transdermal[33] delivery of L-dopa is an interesting option, but the former may be technically challenging. The role of gastric electrical stimulation has not been defined in this population.

Megacolon, acute and chronic

Whereas obstruction of any cause must be included in the differential diagnosis of megacolon, fecal impaction must be high on the list in the patient with neurologic disease and chronic constipation, especially if immobile and in the context of sensory impairment. Plain abdominal radiography may be the only essential investigation. Typically, there is dilatation of the cecum and ascending and transverse colon with less gaseous distention in the left colon. If obstruction needs to be ruled out, nowadays computerized abdominal tomography may be the best option, with barium enema and colonoscopy as alternatives. If colonoscopy is contemplated, the endoscopist needs to be mindful of the risk of a cecal perforation due to the closed loop phenomenon, if obstruction is complete.

The first step in the management of acute megacolon is to search for and, where possible, treat any underlying contributing factor such as medication (eg, baclofen), electrolyte imbalance, sepsis, and, of course, recent surgery. Many cases will resolve spontaneously as the associated primary disorder improves; patient positioning may also promote resolution. In resistant cases, therapy should begin with a pharmacologic approach.

Cholinergic agonists are effective: Ponec and colleagues[166] administered neostigmine in a dose of 2 mg intravenously to 11 patients with acute colonic pseudo-obstruction and compared their outcome with that of 10 who received intravenous saline. Ten of the 11 patients who received neostigmine had prompt colonic decompression compared with none of the 10 patients who received placebo. The median time for response was 4 minutes. Two patients who had an initial response to neostigmine required colonoscopic decompression for recurrence of colonic distention; 1 eventually underwent subtotal colectomy. In contrast, 7 patients in the placebo group and the 1 patient in the neostigmine group without an initial response received open-label neostigmine; all achieved colonic decompression. Given the risk of spontaneous perforation with its associated high mortality, colonoscopy has for some time played an important role in the management of patients with megacolon and significant cecal distention.[167–169] By definition the colon will not be prepared in these patients, and the procedure may therefore be technically difficult. An overall success rate in achieving a reduction in cecal diameter of approximately 70% has been reported, but the recurrence rate has been as high as 40%. Some have advocated the placement of a decompression tube at the time of colonoscopy and have reported that this reduces the recurrence rate. This technique involves the placement of a guidewire through the biopsy channel of the colonoscope with the subsequent insertion of the decompression tube over the guidewire, under fluoroscopic control, following withdrawal of the colonoscope. Colonoscopy should be reserved for those for whom conservative therapy fails, in view of its risks in Ogilvie syndrome.

Surgical intervention, and the placement of a tube cecostomy in particular, may become necessary in the patient with megacolon who seems at high risk of perforation and for whom pharmacologic and colonoscopic attempts at decompression have failed. Clearly, surgery will also be necessary in those who unfortunately progress to ischemia or perforation. In all of these situations surgery has been associated with high morbidity and mortality rates. Prevention of acute megacolon will be based on the avoidance, where possible, of those circumstances that may precipitate this event; particular attention should be paid to medications known to induce hypomotility.

Constipation and incontinence

Laxatives continue to be the backbone of constipation management despite an overwhelming volume of rigorous clinical trial data. Whereas a number of prokinetic agents, including cisapride[170] and tagaserod,[171,172] which had been shown to be effective in the management of constipation in the patient with neurologic disease, have been withdrawn because of adverse events, the prokinetic approach continues to attract interest. "Old" compounds, such as pyridostigmine given orally in the maximum tolerated oral dose (180–540 mg daily), have been shown to accelerate colon transit and improve symptoms among patients with autonomic dysfunction and constipation.[173] A "new" agent, mosapride, has also shown efficacy in constipation in relation to PD,[174] and prucalopride, although not yet tested in PD, MS, or ALS, offers promise.[175]

Nonpharmacologic approaches such as magnetic stimulation[176] and abdominal massage[177] have been shown to be effective in treating constipation related to neurogenic bowel dysfunction, and sacral nerve stimulation has demonstrated long-term efficacy in limited studies in chronic constipation.[178] There are also a number of studies documenting successful treatment of constipation in MS by biofeedback.[67,179,180]

The management of constipation in the context of neurogenic bowel dysfunction must include mindfulness of the possibility of precipitating fecal incontinence and soilage.[16,65,181] One approach to this issue is the technique of transanal irrigation.[182] In this technique, water is instilled into the colon and rectum to instigate a regular and controlled evacuation of feces; this approach has been shown to be effective in spinal cord injury and seems an attractive option in chronic neurologic disease.[182] Other approaches to the management of incontinence in this context include biofeedback[180] and sacral nerve stimulation.[183–186]

SUMMARY

Gastrointestinal symptoms are common in the patient with chronic neurologic disease and may loom large in terms of impact on quality of life and on nutrition and mobility. A knowledge of the range of gastrointestinal disorders associated with a given neurologic disease, together with an understanding of the risks and benefits of various therapeutic options and approaches, should aid gastroenterologists in their efforts to contribute to the care of these patients. In most instances a multidisciplinary team (neurologist/neurosurgeon, gastroenterologist, nutritionist, therapist, specialist nurse) aware of the wishes and needs of the family and their carers and mindful of the nature and the natural history of the underlying disease process are best placed to assess and manage these problems.

REFERENCES

1. Goyal RK, Hirano I. Mechanisms of disease: the enteric nervous system. N Engl J Med 1996;334:1106–15.
2. Mayer EA, Gebhart GF. Basic and clinical aspects of visceral hyperalgesia. Gastroenterology 1994;107:271–93.
3. Smithard DG, O'Neill PA, England R, et al. The natural history of dysphagia following a stroke. Dysphagia 1997;12:188–93.

4. Hamdy S, Rothwell JC, Aziz Q, et al. Organization and reorganization of human swallowing motor cortex: implications for recovery after stroke. Clin Sci (Lond) 2000;99:151–7.
5. Hamdy S, Aziz Q, Rothwell JC, et al. Explaining oropharyngeal dysphagia after unilateral stroke. Lancet 1997;350:686–92.
6. Hamdy S, Rothwell JC. Gut feelings about recovery after stroke: the organization and reorganization of human swallowing motor cortex. Trends Neurosci 1998; 21:278–82.
7. Hamdy S, Aziz Q, Rothwell JC, et al. Recovery of swallowing after dysphagic stroke relates to functional reorganization in the intact motor cortex. Gastroenterology 1998;115:1104–12.
8. Hamdy S, Aziz Q, Rothwell JC, et al. The cortical topography of human swallowing musculature in health and disease. Nat Med 1996;2:1217–24.
9. Schaller BJ, Graf R, Jacobs AH. Pathophysiological changes of the gastrointestinal tract in ischemic stroke. Am J Gastroenterol 2006;101:1655–65.
10. Micklefield GH, Jorgensen E, Blaeser I, et al. Esophageal manometric studies in patients with an apoplectic stroke with/without oropharyngeal dysphagia. Dtsch Med Wochenschr 1999;124(9):239–44 [in German].
11. Gordon C, Hewer RL, Wade DT. Dysphagia in acute stroke. Br Med J (Clin Res Ed) 1987;295:411–4.
12. Otegbayo JA, Talabi OA, Akere A, et al. Gastrointestinal complications in stroke survivors. Trop Gastroenterol 2006;27:127–30.
13. Quigley EM. Gastrointestinal dysfunction in Parkinson's disease. Semin Neurol 1996;16:245–50.
14. Jost WH. Gastrointestinal dysfunction in Parkinson's disease. J Neurol Sci 2010; 289:69–73.
15. Gallagher DA, Lees AJ, Schrag A. What are the most important nonmotor symptoms in patients with Parkinson's disease? Mov Disord 2010;25;2493–500.
16. Pfeiffer RF. Gastrointestinal dysfunction in Parkinson's disease. Parkinsonism Relat Disord 2011;17:10–5.
17. Lebouvier T, Chaumette T, Paillusson S, et al. The second brain and Parkinson's disease. Eur J Neurosci 2009;30:735–41.
18. Natale G, Pasquali L, Ruggieri S, et al. Parkinson's disease and the gut: a well known clinical association in need of an effective cure and explanation. Neurogastroenterol Motil 2008;20:741–9.
19. Singaram C, Ashraf W, Gaumnitz EA, et al. Depletion of dopaminergic neurons in the colon in Parkinson's disease. Lancet 1995;346:861–86.
20. Lebouvier T, Neunlist M, Bruley des Varannes S, et al. Colonic biopsies to assess the neuropathology of Parkinson's disease and its relationship with symptoms. PLoS One 2010;5(9):e12728.
21. Ali GN, Wallace KL, Schwartz R, et al. Mechanisms of oral-pharyngeal dysphagia in patients with Parkinson's disease. Gastroenterology 1996;110:383–92.
22. Born LJ, Harned RH, Rikkers LF, et al. Cricopharyngeal dysfunction in Parkinson's disease: role in dysphagia and response to myotomy. Mov Disord 1996;11:53–8.
23. Cersosimo MG, Benarroch EE. Neural control of the gastrointestinal tract: implications for Parkinson disease. Mov Disord 2008;15:1065–75.
24. Edwards L, Pfeiffer RF, Quigley EM, et al. Incidence of gastrointestinal symptoms in Parkinson's disease. Mov Disord 1991;6:151–6.
25. Colosimo C, Morgante L, Antonini A, et al. Non-motor symptoms in atypical and secondary parkinsonism: the PRIAMO study. J Neurol 2010;257:5–14.

26. Djaldetti R, Baron J, Ziv I, et al. Gastric emptying in Parkinson's disease: patients with and without response fluctuations. Neurology 1996;46:1051–4.
27. Hardoff R, Sula M, Tamir A, et al. Gastric emptying time and gastric motility in patients with Parkinson's disease. Mov Disord 2001;16:1041–7.
28. Goetze O, Wieczorek J, Mueller T, et al. Impaired gastric emptying of a solid test meal in patients with Parkinson's disease using 13C-sodium octanoate breath test. Neurosci Lett 2005;375:170–3.
29. Thomaides T, Karapanaayiotides T, Zoukos Y, et al. Gastric emptying after semi-solid food in multiple system atrophy and Parkinson disease. J Neurol 2005;25: 1055–9.
30. Goetze O, Nikodem AB, Wiezcorek J, et al. Predictors of gastric emptying in Parkinson's disease. Neurogastroenterol Motil 2006;18:369–75.
31. Nyholm D, Lennernas H. Irregular gastrointestinal drug absorption in Parkinson's disease. Expert Opin Drug Metab Toxicol 2008;4:193–203.
32. Eggert K, Schrader C, Hahn M, et al. Continuous jejunal levodopa infusion in patients with advanced parkinson disease: practical aspects and outcome of motor and non-motor complications. Clin Neuropharmacol 2008;31:151–66.
33. Steiger M. Constant dopaminergic stimulation by transdermal delivery of dopaminergic drugs: a new treatment paradigm in Parkinson's disease. Eur J Neurol 2008;15:6–15.
34. Kashihara K. Weight loss in Parkinson's disease. J Neurol 2006;253(Suppl 7): VII38–41.
35. Naftali T, Gadoth N, Huberman M, et al. Electrogastrography in patients with Parkinson's disease. Can J Neurol Sci 2005;32:82–6.
36. Chen CL, Lin HH, Chen SY, et al. Utility of electrogastrography in differentiating Parkinson's disease with or without gastrointestinal symptoms: a prospective controlled study. Digestion 2005;71:187–91.
37. Dobbs RJ, Dobbs SM, Weller C, et al. Role of chronic infection and inflammation in the gastrointestinal tract in the etiology and pathogenesis of idiopathic parkinsonism. Part 1: eradication of Helicobacter in the cachexia of idiopathic parkinsonism. Helicobacter 2005;10:267–75.
38. Bjarnason IT, Charlett A, Dobbs RJ, et al. Role of chronic infection and inflammation in the gastrointestinal tract in the etiology and pathogenesis of idiopathic parkinsonism. Part 2: response of facets of clinical idiopathic parkinsonism to Helicobacter pylori eradication. A randomized, double-blind, placebo-controlled efficacy study. Helicobacter 2005;10:276–87.
39. Weller C, Charlett A, Oxlade NL, et al. Role of chronic infection and inflammation in the gastrointestinal tract in the etiology and pathogenesis of idiopathic parkinsonism. Part 3: predicted probability and gradients of severity of idiopathic parkinsonism based H. pylori antibody profile. Helicobacter 2005;10:288–97.
40. Jost WH, Jung G, Schimrigk K. Colonic transit time in idiopathic Parkinson's syndrome. Eur Neurol 1994;34:329–31.
41. Edwards LL, Quigley EM, Harned RK, et al. Characterization of swallowing and defecation in Parkinson's disease. Am J Gastroenterol 1994;89:15–25.
42. Davies KN, King D, Billington D, et al. Intestinal permeability and orocaecal transit time in elderly patients with Parkinson's disease. Postgrad Med J 1997;73:686–8.
43. Sakakibara R, Odaka T, Uchiyama T, et al. Colonic transit time and rectoanal videomanometry in Parkinson's disease. J Neurol Neurosurg Psychiatry 2003;74: 268–72.
44. Gabrielli M, Bonazzi P, Scarpellini E, et al. Prevalence of small intestinal bacterial overgrowth in Parkinson's disease. Mov Disord 2011;26:889–92.

45. Ashraf W, Pfeiffer RF, Quigley EM. Anorectal manometry in the assessment of anorectal function in Parkinson's disease: a comparison with chronic idiopathic constipation. Mov Disord 1994;9:655–63.
46. Ashraf W, Wszolek ZK, Pfeiffer RF, et al. Anorectal function in fluctuating (on-off) Parkinson's disease: evaluation by combined anorectal manometry and electromyography. Mov Disord 1995;10:650–7.
47. Normand MM, Ashraf W, Quigley EM, et al. Simultaneous electromyography and manometry of the anal sphincter in Parkinsonian patients: technical considerations. Muscle Nerve 1996;19:110–1.
48. Edwards LL, Quigley EM, Harned RK, et al. Defecatory function in Parkinson's disease: response to Apomorphine. Ann Neurol 1993;33:490–3.
49. Toepfer M, Schroeder M, Klauser A, et al. Delayed colonic transit times in amyotrophic lateral sclerosis assessed with radio-opaque markers. Eur J Med Res 1997;2:473–6.
50. Toepfer M, Folwaczny C, Klauser A, et al. Gastrointestinal dysfunction in amyotrophic lateral sclerosis. Amyotroph Lateral Scler Other Motor Neuron Disord 1999; 1:15–9.
51. Carvalho M, Schwartz MS, Swash M. Involvement of the external anal sphincter in amyotrophic lateral sclerosis. Muscle Nerve 1995;18:848–53.
52. Sakuta M, Nakanishi T, Toyokura Y. Anal muscle electromyograms differ in amyotrophic lateral sclerosis and Shy-Drager syndrome. Neurology 1978;28:1289–93.
53. Sumelahti ML, Hakama M, Elovaara I, et al. Causes of death among patients with multiple sclerosis. Mult Scler 2010;16:1437–42.
54. Poorjavad M, Derakhshandeh F, Etemadifar M, et al. Oropharyngeal dysphagia in multiple sclerosis. Mult Scler 2010;16:362–5.
55. Restivo DA, Marchese-Ragona R, Patti F, et al. Botulinum toxin improves dysphagia associated with multiple sclerosis. Eur J Neurol 2011;18:486–90.
56. El-Maghraby TA, Shalaby NM, Al-Tawdy MH, et al. Gastric motility dysfunction in patients with multiple sclerosis assessed by gastric emptying scintigraphy. Can J Gastroenterol 2005;19:141–5.
57. Gupta YK. Gastroparesis with multiple sclerosis. JAMA 1984;252:42.
58. Read SJ, Leggett BA, Pender MP. Gastroparesis with multiple sclerosis. Lancet 1995;346:1228.
59. Raghav S, Kipp D, Watson J, et al. Gastroparesis in multiple sclerosis. Mult Scler 2006;12:243–4.
60. Reddymasu SC, Bonino J, McCallum RW. Gastroparesis secondary to a demyelinating disease: a case series. BMC Gastroenterol 2007;7:3.
61. Ben-Zvi JS, Daniel SJ. Painless gastric perforation in a patient with multiple sclerosis. Am J Gastroenterol 1988;83:1008–11.
62. Haensch CA, Jorg J. Autonomic dysfunction in multiple sclerosis. J Neurol 2006; 253(Suppl 1):I3–9.
63. Fowler CJ, Henry MM. Gastrointestinal dysfunction in multiple sclerosis. Semin Neurol 1996;16:277–9.
64. Norton C, Chelvanayagam S. Bowel problems and coping strategies in people with multiple sclerosis. Br J Nurs 2010;19:221–6.
65. Winge K, Rasmussen D, Werdein LM. Constipation in neurological diseases. J Neurol Neurosurg Psychiatry 2003;74:13–9.
66. Krogh K, Christensen P. Neurogenic colorectal and pelvic floor dysfunction. Best Pract Res Clin Gastroenterol 2009;23:531–43.

67. Munteis E, Andreu M, Martinez-Rodriguez J, et al. Manometric correlations of anorectal dysfunction and biofeedback outcome in patients with multiple sclerosis. Mult Scler 2008;14:237–42.
68. Chia YW, Gill KP, Jameson JS, et al. Paradoxical puborectalis contraction is a feature of constipation in patients with multiple sclerosis. J Neurol Neurosurg Psychiatry 1996;60:31–5.
69. Quigley EM. The pathophysiology of diabetic gastroenteropathy: more vague than vagal. Gastroenterology 1997;115:1790–4.
70. He CL, Soffer EE, Ferris CD, et al. Loss of interstitial cells of cajal and inhibitory innervation in insulin-dependent diabetes. Gastroenterology 2001;121:427–34.
71. Kempler P, Amarenco G, Freeman R, et al on behalf of the Toronto Consensus panel on Diabetic Neuropathy. Gastrointestinal autonomic neuropathy, erectile-, bladder- and sudomotor dysfunction in patients with diabetes mellitus: clinical impact, assessment, diagnosis and management. Diabetes Metab Res Rev 2011;July 11 [Epub ahead of print].
72. Freeman R. Autonomic peripheral neuropathy. Lancet 2005;365:1259–70.
73. Klein CM, Vernino S, Lennon VA, et al. The spectrum of autoimmune autonomic neuropathies. Ann Neurol 2003;53:752–8.
74. Koike H, Atsuta N, Adachi H, et al. Clinicopathological features of acute autonomic and sensory neuropathy. Brain 2010;133:2881–96.
75. Van Doorn PA, Ruts L, Jacobs BC. Clinical features, pathogenesis, and treatment of Guillain-Barré syndrome. Lancet Neurol 2008;7:939–50.
76. Pithadia AB, Kakadia N. Guillain-Barré syndrome (GBS). Pharmacol Rep 2010;62: 220–32.
77. McDougall AJ, McLeod JG. Autonomic neuropathy, I. Clinical features, investigation, pathophysiology, and treatment. J Neurol Sci 1996;137:79–88.
78. Sivadon-Tardy V, Orlokowski D, Rozenberg F, et al. Guillain-Barré syndrome, greater Paris area. Emerg Infect Dis 2006;12:990–3.
79. Aarli JA. Oculopharyngeal muscular dystrophy. Acta Neurol Scand 1969;45: 485–92.
80. Munitz V, Ortiz A, Martinez de Haro LF, et al. Diagnosis and treatment of oculopharyngeal dystrophy: a report of three cases from the same family. Dis Esophagus 2003;16:160–4.
81. Simpson AJ, Khilnani MT. Gastrointestinal manifestations of the muscular dystrophies. Am J Roentgenol Radium Ther Nucl Med 1975;125:948–55.
82. Nowak TV, Ionasescu V, Anuras S. Gastrointestinal manifestations of the muscular dystrophies. Gastroenterology 1982;82:800–10.
83. Karasick D, Karasick S, Mapp E. Gastrointestinal radiologic manifestations of proximal spinal muscular atrophy (Kugelberg-Welander syndrome). J Natl Med Assoc 1982;74:475–8.
84. Staiano A, Del Giudice E, Romano A, et al. Upper gastrointestinal tract motility in children with progressive muscular dystrophy. J Pediatr 1992;121:720–4.
85. Bellini M, Biagi S, Stasi S, et al. Gastrointestinal manifestations in myotonic muscular dystrophy. World J Gastroenterol 2006;12:1821–8.
86. Ronnblom A, Forsberg H, Danielsson A. Gastrointestinal symptoms in myotonic dystrophy. Scand J Gastroenterol 1996;31:654–7.
87. Tieleman AA, van Vliet J, Jansen JBMJ, et al. Gastrointestinal involvement is frequent in Myotonic Dystrophy type 2. Neuromuscular Disord 2008;18:646–9.
88. Swick HM, Werlin SL, Dodds WJ, et al. Pharyngoesophageal motor function in patients with myotonic dystrophy. Ann Neurol 1981;10:454–7.

89. Bellini M, Alduini P, Costa F, et al. Gastric emptying in myotonic dystrophy patients. Dig Liver Dis 2002;34:484–8.
90. Ronnblom A, Andersson S, Hellstrom PM, et al. Gastric emptying in myotonic dystrophy. Eur J Clin Invest 2002;32:570–4.
91. Horowitz M, Maddox A, Maddern GJ, et al. Gastric and esophageal emptying in dystrophia myotonica. Effect of metoclopramide. Gastroenterology 1987;92:570–7.
92. Lewis TD, Daniel EE. Gastroduodenal motility in a case of dystrophia myotonica. Gastroenterology 1981;81:145–9.
93. Nowak TV, Anuras S, Brown BP, et al. Small intestinal motility in myotonic dystrophy patients. Gastroenterology 1984;86:808–13.
94. Bruinenberg JF, Rieu PN, Gabreels FM, et al. Intestinal pseudo-obstruction syndrome in a child with myotonic dystrophy. Acta Paediatr 1996;85:121–3.
95. Brunner HG, Hamel BCJ, Rieu P, et al. Intestinal pseudo-obstruction in myotonic dystrophy. J Med Genet 1992;29:791–3.
96. Abercrombie JF, Rogers J, Swash M. Faecal incontinence in myotonic dystrophy. J Neurol Neurosurg Psychiatry 1998;64:128–30.
97. Lecointe-Besancon I, Leroy F, Devroede G, et al. A comparative study of esophageal and anorectal motility in myotonic dystrophy. Dig Dis Sci 1999;44:1090–9.
98. Kusunoki M, Hatada T, Ikeuchi H, et al. Gastric volvulus complicating myotonic dystrophy. Hepatogastroenterology 1992;39:586–8.
99. Torretta A, Mascagni D, Zeri KP, et al. The megacolon in myotonic dystrophy: case report and review of the literature. Ann Ital Chir 2000;71:729–32 [in Italian].
100. Jaffe KM, McDonald CM, Ingman E, et al. Symptoms of upper gastrointestinal dysfunction in Duchenne muscular dystrophy: case-control study. Arch Phys Med Rehabil 1990;71:742–4.
101. Pane M, Vasta I, Messina S, et al. Feeding problems and weight gain in Duchenne muscular dystrophy. Eur J Paediatr Neurol 2006;10:231–6.
102. Camelo AL, Awad RA, Madrazo A, et al. Esophageal motility disorders in Mexican patients with Duchenne's muscular dystrophy. Acta Gastroenterol Latinoam 1997; 27:119–22.
103. Borrelli O, Salvia G, Mancini V, et al. Evolution of gastric electrical features and gastric emptying in children with Duchenne and Becker muscular dystrophy. Am J Gastroenterol 2005;100:695–702.
104. Barohn RJ, Levine EJ, Olson JO, et al. Gastric hypomotiltiy in Duchenne's muscular dystrophy. N Engl J Med 1988;319:15–8.
105. Bensen ES, Jaffe KM, Tarr PI. Acute gastric dilatation in Duchenne muscular dystrophy: a case report and review of the literature. Arch Phys Med Rehabil 1996;77:512–4.
106. Chung BC, Park HJ, Yoon SB, et al. Acute gastroparesis in Duchenne's muscular dystrophy. Yonsei Med J 1998;39:175–9.
107. Korman SH, Bar-Oz B, Granot E, et al. Orocaecal transit time in Duchenne muscular dystrophy. Arch Dis Child 1991;66:143–4.
108. Leon SH, Schuffler MD, Kettler M, et al. Chronic intestinal pseudoobstruction as a complication of Duchenne's muscular dystrophy. Gastroenterology 1986;90:455–9.
109. Drachman DB. Myasthenia gravis. N Engl J Med 1994;330:1797–810.
110. Anderson NE, Hutchinson DO, Nicholson GJ, et al. Intestinal pseudo-obstruction, myasthenia gravis, and thymoma. Neurology 1996;47:985–7.
111. Priefer BA, Robbins J. Eating changes in mild-stage Alzheimer's disease: a pilot study. Dysphagia 1997;12:212–21.
112. O'Mahony D, O'Leary P, Quigley EM. Aging and intestinal motility: a review of factors that affect intestinal motility in the aged. Drugs Aging 2002;19:515–27.

113. Sonnenberg A, Tsou VT, Muller AD. The "institutional colon": a frequent colonic dysmotility in psychiatric and neurologic disease. Am J Gastroenterol 1994;89: 62–6.
114. Kahrilas PJ. Swallowing disorders. In: Quigley EM, Pfeiffer RF, editors. Neurogastroenterology. Philadelphia: Butterworth Heinemann; 2004. p. 147–62.
115. Smithard DG, O'Neill PA, Park C, et al,Northwest Dysphagia Group. Can bedside assessment reliably exclude aspiration following acute stroke? Age Ageing 1998;27: 99–106.
116. Smithard DG, O'Neill PA, Park C, et al. Complications and outcomes after acute stroke. Does dysphagia matter? Stroke 1996;27:1200–4.
117. Tougas G, Eaker EY, Abell TL, et al. Assessment of gastric emptying using a low fat meal: establishment of international control values. Am J Gastroenterol 2000;95: 1456–62.
118. Rao SS, Kuo B, McCallum RW, et al. Investigation of colonic and whole-gut transit with wireless motility capsule and radiopaque markers in constipation. Clin Gastroenterol Hepatol 2009;7:537–44.
119. Parkman HP, Camilleri M, Farrugia G, et al. Gastroparesis and functional dyspepsia: excerpts from the AGA/ANMS meeting. Neurogastroenterol Motil 2010;22:113–33.
120. Quigley EM. Acute intestinal pseudo-obstruction. Curr Treat Opt Gastroenterol 2000;3:273–85.
121. Odunsi ST, Camilleri M. Selected interventions in nuclear medicine: gastrointestinal motor functions. Semin Nucl Med 2009;39:186–94.
122. Camilleri M, Bharucha AE, di Lorenzo C, et al. American Neurogastroenterology and Motility Society consensus statement on intraluminal measurement of gastrointestinal and colonic motility in clinical practice. Neurogastroenterol Motil 2008;20:1269–82.
123. Tantiphlachiva K, Rao P, Attaluri A, et al. Digital rectal examination is a useful tool for identifying patients with dyssynergia. Clin Gastroenterol Hepatol 2010;8:955–60.
124. Bharucha AE, Fletcher JG. Recent advances in assessing anorectal structure and functions. Gastroenterology 2007;133:1069–74.
125. Jones MP, Post J, Crowell MD. High-resolution manometry in the evaluation of anorectal disorders: a simultaneous comparison with water-perfused manometry. Am J Gastroenterol 2007;102:850–5.
126. Rasley A, Logemann JA, Kahrilas PJ, et al. Prevention of barium aspiration during video fluoroscopic swallowing studies: value of change in posture. AJR Am J Roentgenol 1993;160:1005–9.
127. Kahrilas PJ, Logemann JA, Krugler C, et al. Volitional augmentation of upper esophageal sphincter opening during swallowing. Am J Physiol 1991;260:G450–6.
128. Giusti A, Giambuzzi M. Management of dysphagia in patients affected by multiple sclerosis: state of the art. Neurol Sci 2008;29:S364–6.
129. Wood LD, Neumiller JJ, Setter SM, et al. Clinical review of treatment options for select nonmotor symptoms of Parkinson's disease. Am J Geriatr Pharmacother 2010;8:294–315.
130. Mitchell SL, Tetroe JM. Survival after percutaneous endoscopic gastrostomy placement in older persons. J Gerontol A Biol Sci Med Sci 2000;55:M735–9.
131. Finucane TE, Christmas C, Travis K. Tube feeding in patients with advanced dementia: a review of the evidence. JAMA 1999;282:1365–70.
132. Royal College of Physicians. Oral feeding difficulties and dilemmas: a guide to practical care particularly towards the end of life. London: Royal College of Physicians; 2010.

133. Mitchell SL, Teno JM, Roy J, et al. Clinical and organizational factors associated with feeding tube use among nursing home residents with advanced cognitive impairment. JAMA 2003;290:73–80.
134. Hoffer LJ. Tube feeding in advanced dementia: the metabolic perspective. BMJ 2006;333:1214–5.
135. Ansell P. Thank you. BMJ 2007;334:8.
136. Sampson EL, Candy B, Jones L. Enteral tube feeding for older people with advanced dementia. Cochrane Database Syst Rev 2009;2:CD007209.
137. Dennis MS, Lewis SC, Warlow C. Effect of timing and method of enteral tube feeding for dysphagic stroke patients (FOOD): a multicentre randomized controlled trial. Lancet 2005;365:764–72.
138. Finucane TE, Bynum JP. Use of tube feeding to prevent aspiration pneumonia. Lancet 1996;348(9039):1421–4.
139. Balan KK, Vinjamuri S, Maltby P et al. Gastroesophageal reflux in patients fed by percutaneous endoscopic gastrostomy (PEG): detection by a simple scintigraphic method. Am J Gastroenterol 1998;93:946–9.
140. Miller RG, Jackson CE, Kasarskis EJ, et al. Practice parameter update: the care of the patient with amyotrophic lateral sclerosis: drug, nutritional, and respiratory therapies (an evidence-based review). Neurology 2009;73:1218–26.
141. Desport JC, Mabrouk T, Bouillet P, et al. Complications and survival following radiologically and endoscopically-guided gastrostomy in patients with amyotrophic lateral sclerosis. Amyotroph Lateral Scler Other Motor Neuron Disord 2005;6:88–93.
142. Quigley EM. Gastric motor and sensory function and motor disorders of the stomach. In: Feldman F, Friedman LS, Brandt LE, et al, editors. Gastrointestinal and liver disease. pathophysiology/diagnosis/management. 8th edition. Philadelphia: WB Saunders Co; 2002. p. 691–713.
143. Gentilcore D, O'Donovan D, Jones KL, et al. Nutrition therapy for diabetic gastroparesis. Curr Diab Rep 2003;3:418–26.
144. Felsher J, Chand B, Ponsky J. Decompressive percutaneous endoscopic gastroscopy in nonmalignant disease. Am J Surg 2004;187:254–6.
145. Ladas SD, Triantafyllou K, Tzathas C, et al. Gastric phytobezoars may be treated by Coca-Cola lavage. Eur J Gastroenterol Hepatol 2002;14:801–3.
146. Quigley EM. Pharmacotherapy of gastroparesis. Expert Opin Pharmacother 2000; 1:881–7.
147. Camilleri M, Talley NJ. Pathophysiology as a basis for understanding symptom correlates and therapeutic targets. Neurogastroenterol Motil 2004;16:135–42.
148. Friedenberg F, Gullamudi G, Parkman HP. The use of botulinum toxin for the treatment of gastrointestinal motility disorders. Dig Dis Sci 2004;49:165–75.
149. Ezzeddine D, Jit R, Katz M, et al. Pyloric injection of botulinum toxin for treatment of diabetic gastroparesis. Gastrointest Endosc 2002;55:920–3.
150. Lacy BE, Zayat EM, Crowell MD, et al. Botulinum toxin for the treatment of gastroparesis: a preliminary report. Am J Gastroenterol 2002;97:1548–52.
151. Miller LS, Szych GA, Kantor SB, et al. Treatment of idiopathic gastroparesis with injection of botulinum toxin in to the pyloric sphincter muscle. Am J Gastroenterol 2002;97:1653–60.
152. Gupta P, Rao SS. Attenuation of isolated pyloric pressure waves in gastroparesis in response to botulinum toxin injection: a case report. Gastrointest Endosc 2002;56: 770–2.
153. McCallum RW, Chen JDZ, Lin Z, et al. Gastric pacing improves emptying and symptoms in patients with gastroparesis. Gastroenterology 1998;114:456–61.

154. Familoni BO, Abell TL, Voeller G, et al. Electrical stimulation at a frequency higher than basal rate in human stomach. Dig Dis Sci 1997;42:885–91.
155. Abell TL, Van Cutsem E, Abrahamsson H, et al. Gastric electrical stimulation in intractable symptomatic gastroparesis. Digestion 2002;66:204–12.
156. Abell T, Lou J, Tabbaa M, et al. Gastric electrical stimulation for gastroparesis improves nutritional parameters at short, intermediate, and long-term follow up. JPEN J Parenter Enteral Nutr 2003;27:277–81.
157. Lin Z, Forster J, Sarosiek I, et al. Treatment of diabetic gastroparesis by high-frequency gastric electrical stimulation. Diabetes Care 2004;27:1071–6.
158. Luo J, Al-Juburi A, Rashed H, et al. Gastric electrical stimulation is associated with improvement in pancreatic endocrine function in humans. Pancreas 2004;29: e41–4.
159. Abell TL, McCallum R, Hocking M, et al. Gastric electrical stimulation for medically refractory gastroparesis. Gastroenterology 2003;125:421–8.
160. Tougas G, Huizinga JD. Gastric pacing as a treatment for intractable gastroparesis—shocking news? Gastroenterology 1998;114:598–601.
161. Hannon MJ, Dinneen S, Yousif O, et al. Gastric pacing for diabetic gastroparesis–does it work? Ir Med J 2011;104:135–7.
162. Becker JC, Dietl KH, Konturek JW, et al. Gastric wall perforation: a rare complication of gastric electrical stimulation. Gastrointest Endosc 2004;59:584–6.
163. Ejskjaer NT, Bradley JL, Buxton-Thomas MS, et al. Novel surgical treatment and gastric pathology in diabetic gastroparesis. Diabet Med 1999;16:488–95.
164. Watkins PJ, Buxton-Thomas MS, Howard ER. Long-term outcome after gastrectomy for intractable diabetic gastroparesis. Diabet Med 2003;20:58–63.
165. Jones MP, Maganti K. A systematic review of surgical therapy for gastroparesis. Am J Gastroenterol 2003;98:2122–9.
166. Ponec RJ, Saunders MD, Kimmey MB. Neostigmine for the treatment of acute colonic pseudo-obstruction. New Eng J Med 1999;341:137–41.
167. Strodel WE, Brothers T. Colonoscopic decompression of pseudo-obstruction and volvulus. Surg Clin North Am 1989;69:1327–35.
168. Rex DK. Colonoscopy and acute colonic pseudo-obstruction. Gastrointest Endosc Clin North Am 1997;7:499–508.
169. Laine L. Management of acute colonic pseudo-obstruction. New Eng J Med 1999;341:192–3.
170. Quigley EM. Cisapride: what can we learn from the rise and fall of a prokinetic? J Dig Dis 2011;12:147–56.
171. Sullivan KL, Staffetti JF, Hauser RA, et al. Tegaserod (Zelnorm) for the treatment of constipation in Parkinson's disease. Mov Disord 2006;21:115–6.
172. Morgan JC, Sethi KD. Tegaserod in constipation associated with Parkinson's disease. Clin Neuropharmacol 2007;30:52–4.
173. Bharucha AE, Low PA, Camilleri M, et al. Pilot study of pyridostigmine in constipated patients with autonomic neuropathy. Clin Auton Res 2008;18:194–202.
174. Liu Z, Sakakibara R, Odaka T, et al. Mosapride citrate, a novel 5-HT4 agonist and partial 5-HT3 antagonist, ameliorates constipation in parkinsonian patients. Mov Disord 2005;20:680–6.
175. Quigley EM. Prucalopride: safety, efficacy and potential applications. Therap Adv Gastroenterol 2011, in press.
176. Tsai PY, Wang CP, Chiu FY, et al. Efficacy of functional magnetic stimulation in neurogenic bowel dysfunction after spinal cord injury. J Rehabil Med 2009;41:41–7.

177. McClurg D, Hagen S, Hawkins S, et al. Abdominal massage for the alleviation of constipation symptoms in people with multiple sclerosis: a randomized controlled feasibility study. Mult Scler 2011;17:223–33.
178. Kamm MA, Dudding TC, Melenhorst J, et al. Sacral nerve stimulation for intractable constipation. Gut 2010;59:333–40.
179. Preziosi G, Raptis DA, Storrie J, et al. Bowel biofeedback treatment in patients with multiple sclerosis and bowel symptoms. Dis Colon Rectum 2011;54:1114–21.
180. Wiesel PH, Norton C, Roy AJ, et al. Gut focused behavioural treatment (biofeedback) for constipation and faecal incontinence in multiple sclerosis. J Neurol Neurosurg Psychiatry 2000;69:240–3.
181. DasGupta R, Fowler CJ. Bladder, bowel and sexual dysfunction in multiple sclerosis: management strategies. Drugs 2003;63:153–66.
182. Emmanuel A. Review of the efficacy and safety of transanal irrigation for neurogenic bowel dysfunction. Spinal Cord 2010;48:664–73.
183. Matzel KE, Kamm MA, Stösser M, et al. Sacral spinal nerve stimulation for faecal incontinence: multicentre study. Lancet 2004;363:1270–6.
184. Jarrett ME, Matzel KE, Christiansen J, et al. Sacral nerve stimulation for faecal incontinence in patients with previous partial spinal injury including disc prolapse. Br J Surg 2005;92:734–9.
185. Jarrett ME, Mowatt G, Glazener CM, et al. Systematic review of sacral nerve stimulation for faecal incontinence and constipation. Br J Surg 2004;91:1559–69.
186. Gourcerol G, Gallas S, Michot F, et al. Sacral nerve stimulation in fecal incontinence: are there factors associated with success? Dis Colon Rectum 2007;50:3–12.

Motility Problems in the Intellectually Challenged Child, Adolescent, and Young Adult

Massimo Martinelli, MD, Annamaria Staiano, MD*

KEYWORDS

- Gastrointestinal motility disorders • Down syndrome
- Cerebral palsy • Familial dysautonomia • Williams syndrome

DOWN SYNDROME

Down syndrome (DS) is the most common chromosomal abnormality occurring in humans. In Europe, DS accounts for 8% of all registered cases of congenital anomalies. Throughout the world, the overall prevalence of DS is 10 per 10,000 live births, although in recent years this figure has been increasing. DS is characterized by several dysmorphic features, delayed psychomotor development, and low muscle tone in early infancy.[1] DS is associated with dysfunctions that might affect almost every organ and system, including the gut. It has been reported that more than 77% of DS affected neonates have, or develop, associated gastrointestinal (GI) disorders.[2] These conditions can be classified into mechanical and functional disorders and can be primary or secondary.

Next to the most common associated congenital malformations, such as tracheo–esophageal fistula, duodenal atresia/stenosis, and imperforate anus, the most frequently occurring GI disorders in DS are characterized by motor disturbances, particularly encountered in the esophagus and colon. DS affected infants have been reported to be at 100-fold increased risk for Hirschsprung disease (HSCRD). In addition, gastroesophageal reflux disease (GERD), achalasia, and unexplained chronic constipation often complicate the clinical course of DS children.[3] According to a recent report by Van Trotsenburg and colleagues, GI disorders and feeding difficulties represent a very frequent cause of hospitalization (19%) in patients affected by DS.[4] Unfortunately, the inherent difficulties of DS patients to express themselves could hamper clinical evaluation and delay the diagnosis, increasing the

The authors have nothing to disclose.
Department of Pediatrics, University of Naples "Federico II," Via Pansini No. 5, 80131, Naples, Italy
* Corresponding author.
E-mail address: staiano@unina.it

Gastroenterol Clin N Am 40 (2011) 765–775
doi:10.1016/j.gtc.2011.09.009

risk of related complications. The likelihood of the involvement of the enteric nervous system (ENS) in these associations, although not yet completely understood, is generally accepted.

Role of the Enteric Nervous System

The anomalous central nervous system (CNS) development, function, and intellectual impairment in DS has always been related to the genetic imbalance, resulting from the presence of an extra copy of chromosome 21. However, the underlying pathogenetic mechanisms are still unclear. Whether chromosome 21 trisomy determines a malfunction of dosage-sensitive genes or results in a more generalized alteration of homeostasis in a critical development period is still not clarified.[3] In this context, it is not surprising to observe a high frequency of enteric nervous system alterations, as both embryonic brain and GI tract development are regulated by similar neural growth factors, under the control of the same genes. A link between brain and ENS development is well demonstrated by the high prevalence of cerebral dysgenesis in patients affected by neurocristopathies, such as HSCRD.[5] The ENS develops from the colonization of neural crest cells, which migrate to populate the GI tract. This mechanism is regulated by a complex signaling system, which appears to be altered in DS. Decreased neuronal migration, as well as alterations of dendritic development, has been shown in an animal model of DS.[6] At the same time, alterations in ENS structure and function have been demonstrated in DS patients. Nakazato and Landing showed a reduced number of neurons in esophageal plexus ganglia in DS patients.[7] Hypothetically, this decrease, described in the esophagus, could occur throughout the entire gut. Further studies are needed to better clarify these fundamental pathogenetic mechanisms.

Esophageal Motor Dysfunction

In a recent prospective analysis, Zarate and colleagues reported that the most common functional GI symptoms described in DS patients are dysphagia for liquids and solids, vomiting, regurgitation, and heartburn.[8] GERD remains one of the most frequent causes of esophageal symptomatology in DS. Previous studies described a high prevalence of severe GERD with the occurrence of serious complications, such as oropharyngeal aspiration and pneumonia, in 43% of DS patients.[9,10] In one case report, GERD was associated with the development of pulmonary arterial hypertension in a 2-month-old DS-affected boy.[11]

As is the case with all children with a neurologic impairment, many factors could contribute to the high prevalence of reflux and impaired esophageal clearance and, consequently, lead to the development and progression of GERD among DS patients. For example, abnormal swallowing, delayed gastric emptying, abnormal muscle tone, obesity, and constipation are commonly reported in this patient population. The severity of GERD may also result from poor self-protective mechanisms and delayed diagnosis caused by difficulties in obtaining an accurate history of symptoms. In addition, it seems that the severity of GERD correlates directly to the severity of neurologic impairment.[12] For all these reasons it seems extremely important to investigate esophageal function in all patients with typical or such atypical GERD symptoms as food rejection, frequent vomiting, coughing, and failure to thrive. Early diagnosis is essential to prevent respiratory problems, growth retardation, and all other GERD complications. According to the latest European Society for Pediatric Gastroenterology, Hepatology, and Nutrition (ESPGHAN)–North American Society for Pediatric Gastroenterology, Hepatology, and Nutrition (NASPGHAN) guidelines on GERD, the evaluation of children with neurologic impairment, such as DS, should be

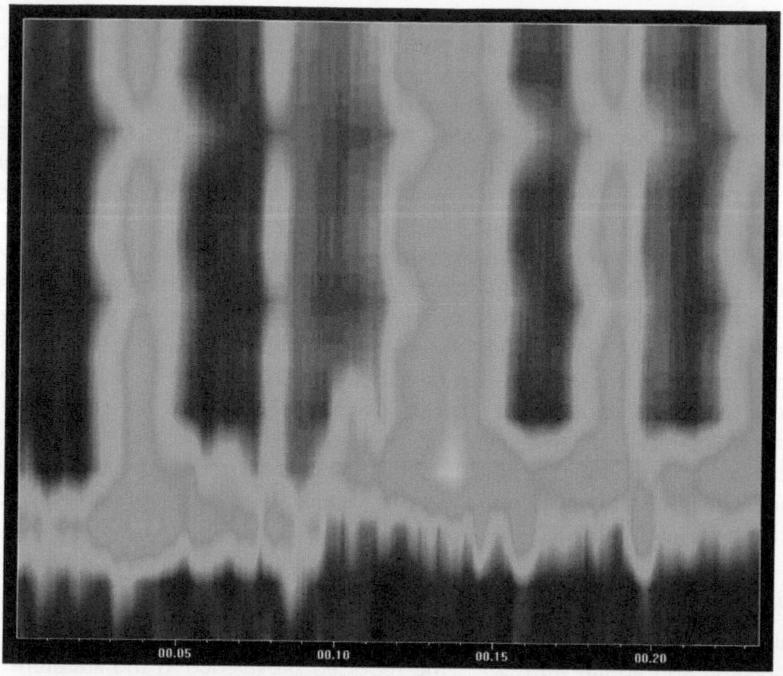

Fig. 1. Example of achalasia. High-resolution manometry tracing in a patient affected by DS. Note a complete absence of peristaltic sequences. The peristaltic sequence is replaced by isobaric contour stripes spanning the esophageal body.

based on a high index of suspicion and must not only confirm the diagnosis but also rule out alternative diagnoses. Contrast GI radiographic studies, upper GI endoscopy and biopsy, metabolic and drug toxicity screening, and pH/impedance studies may be required.[12] Treatment should associate optimized antisecretory therapy to behavioral measures, including feeding and positional changes. Given the morbidity and high failure rates of antireflux surgery, patients whose symptoms are well controlled on medical therapy may not derive additional benefit from antireflux surgery.[12] Despite optimized medical therapy, some DS patients affected by GERD need antireflux surgery. However, this should be considered only in highly selected cases, as antireflux surgery has been independently associated with poorer developmental outcome.[4] In addition, it has been shown that preexisting esophageal dysmotility in DS patients could complicate the postoperative clinical course after corrective surgical procedures.[13]

Next to GERD, esophageal motor disorders, such as achalasia, are not infrequent in DS patients. A number of instances of the association between achalasia and DS have been described in adult and pediatric DS populations[14,15] (**Fig. 1**). In a study conducted by Zarate and colleagues, the authors evaluated esophageal clearance in adult DS patients and controls, using scintigraphy. Patients with abnormal scintigraphic studies and suggestive symptoms proceeded to undergo radiologic and manometric examinations.[8] Results clearly showed a significantly greater retention of both liquid and semisolid boluses in DS. Achalasia was diagnosed in two patients, providing an astonishingly high prevalence (2/58 patients enrolled) compared with the general population (prevalence 8/100,000).[8] Further, another patient had total body aperistalsis and two had a nonspecific motor disorder. The same authors, in 1999, reported five cases of DS associated with achalasia. Two of the five reported cases were children.[16] Why does DS carry a higher risk of achalasia?

Achalasia is a primary esophageal disorder of unknown etiology: infectious, autoimmune, and genetic factors have been implicated.[17] Although the increased susceptibility of DS patients to infection, as well as their predilection to autoimmune disorders, could be the link between these disorders, genetic factors and associated alterations of ENS morphology and function probably play the most important role.[8] HSCRD, another primary congenital disorder, is also more prevalent in DS. Both achalasia and HSCRD share some pathophysiologic mechanisms, such as a lack of nitric oxide synthase in the affected region, a reduced number of ganglion cells in affected regions, and a consequent failure of sphincter relaxation.[18,19] Symptoms in pediatric patients with achalasia can be subtle and, in contrast to adults, dysphagia is not always present. Indeed, the main clinical features are respiratory symptoms and growth retardation.[16] In any event, an early diagnosis of achalasia is extremely important in childhood and achalasia should always be included with GERD in the differential diagnosis of any esophageal or potentially esophageal-related symptoms in pediatric patients with DS.

Unexplained Chronic Constipation and HSCRD

Chronic constipation remains one of the most common symptoms experienced by both children and adults with DS[14]: the reported prevalence in the literature varies from 19% to 56%. Further, these rates may represent an underestimate. All DS children with constipation must be considered to be potential candidates for HSCRD, because of the known association between these two entities. HSCRD remains the most common congenital dysganglionosis associated with DS. Reported incidence is approximately one in 200 to 300 DS patients, higher than the 0.15% to 0.17% expected incidence in the general population.[20] Looking at it from another perspective, about 30% of HSCRD patients have a recognized chromosomal abnormality, syndrome, or additional congenital anomalies, the most frequent of which is DS.[21] This well described association has led to the proposal that chromosome 21 may play a possible role in the pathogenesis of HSCRD. Nevertheless, although the presence of trisomy 21 seems to be associated with a higher risk for the disorder, it does not invariably lead to HSCRD. Several studies have investigated the role of chromosome 21 as a potential candidate area, capable of modifying the risk of HSCRD.[22] Possible relationships between DS and major susceptibility HSCRD genes, such as *RET* and *EDNRB*, have also been examined. Arnold and colleagues showed that the *RET* enhancer polymorphism RET +9.7 correlates with HSCRD in DS.[23] At the same time, a novel *EDNRB* variant has been identified in DS patients with HSCRD.[24]

Although the precise pathogenesis of HSCRD in DS has yet to be clarified, HSCRD should always be considered in DS patients. Moore reported a prevalence of 3.2%, with a female preponderance and an 85% rate of other associated anomalies. The aganglionic segment was limited in extent to the rectosigmoid in 69% of cases.[25] Early diagnosis is extremely important owing to the high reported mortality. DS patients show a significantly higher overall risk of preoperative and postoperative enterocolitis.[26] These inferior outcomes could be explained by an impaired immunologic response.[27,28] In addition, long-term outcome may also be inferior, as DS patients with HSCRD appear to have a less predictable prognosis.[29] Thus, previous studies reported persisting soiling after the fourth year of life in 60% of patients.[20]

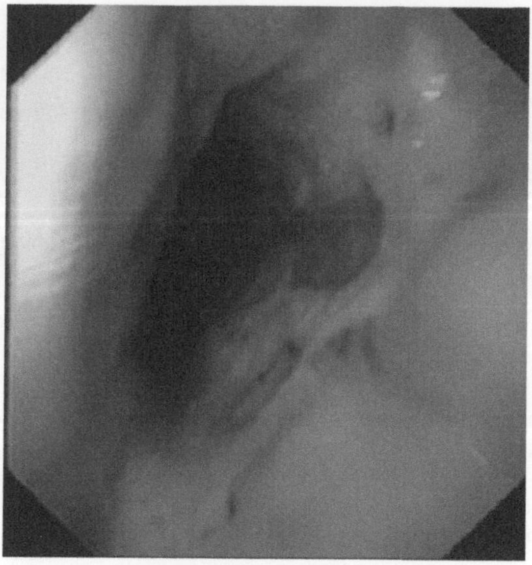

Fig. 2. Severe esophagitis in a child affected by cerebral palsy.

CEREBRAL PALSY

Cerebral palsy refers to a group of chronic, nonprogressive disorders of movement, posture, and tone due to CNS damage before cerebral development is complete. The availability of neonatal intensive care units and high-technology diagnostic procedures has led to an increased survival rate for premature and term infants with neurologic impairment. The prevalence of cerebral palsy is estimated to be 2 per 1000 live births. The relative prevalence of the different types of cerebral palsy varies from series to series, with the spastic type considered to be the most frequent, while periventricular leukomalacia and cortical/cerebral atrophy represent the most typical neuropathologic substrates.[30] GI motor dysfunctions, such as GERD, dysphagia, vomiting, and chronic constipation, have all been reported in children with different degrees of CNS damage. The degree of GI dysmotility seems to correlate with the degree of brain damage.[31] The long-term survival of children with severe neurologic damage, such as cerebral palsy, has created a major challenge for medical care.

Esophageal Dysfunction

GERD is very common in patients with severe neurologic impairment. The incidence, in various studies, has been reported to be between 70% and 90%, depending in part, on the method of investigation, whether using esophageal pH studies or upper GI endoscopy.[32,33] In 1999, our group clearly showed that neurologic patients affected by GERD had delayed gastric emptying and abnormal esophageal motility.[33] This suggests that impaired GI motility is the main pathogenetic factor in the induction and progression of GERD, as well as of severe esophagitis (**Fig. 2**). The main motor abnormalities consisted of significantly lower amplitude of both lower esophageal sphincter (LES) pressure and esophageal body contractions and an increased number of simultaneous waves, compared to control children[33] (**Fig. 3**). These findings, coupled with spasticity, prolonged adoption of supine position, scoliosis, seizures, and a reduction in the amount of swallowed saliva consequent upon

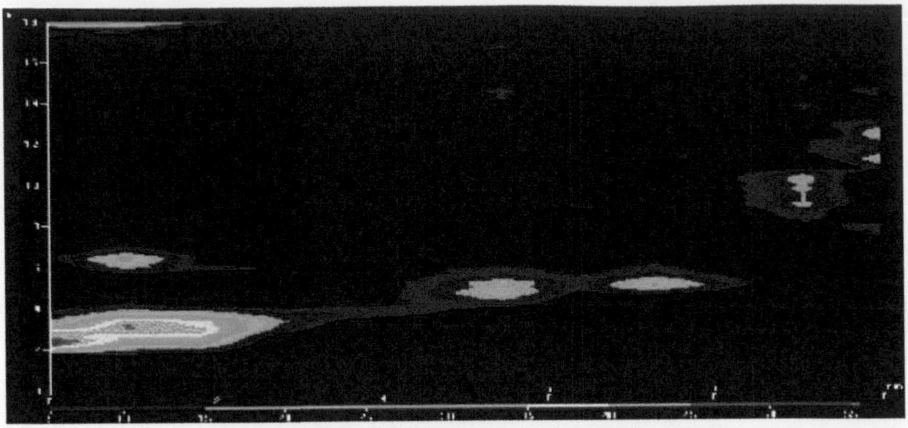

Fig. 3. Example of a high-resolution esophageal manometry tracing in a child affected by cerebral palsy. Note hypocontractility of the distal esophagus with evidence of two distal segments, each of low amplitude. The third segment is foreshortened, extending to the region of the third pressure trough proximal to lower sphincter after contraction.

drooling, increase the predisposition to the development of GERD and may be responsible for the high failure rate of both medical and surgical treatment approaches to this category of patients. Indeed, the optimal management approach to GERD in patients with brain damage is still controversial. According to the recent ESPGHAN–NASPGHAN guidelines on gastroesophageal reflux, antisecretory therapy should be optimized.[12] Long-term treatment with proton pump inhibitors (PPIs) is often effective for symptom control and maintenance of remission.[34,35] Baclofen is also recommended to control GERD symptoms and to reduce vomiting.[36,37] Changes in feeding volume, consistency, and frequency, as well as positional changes, may be helpful. An alternative to this classic medical approach is represented by the use of an elemental diet. We reported a lower incidence of GERD in neurologically impaired children with refractory esophagitis treated with an amino-acid–based formula.[38] However, conventional medical management is known to be less effective in neurologically impaired children and often vomiting tends to persist despite PPIs therapy. At the same time, surgical intervention is associated with a high operative risk[39] and the benefit/risk ratio for antireflux surgery in these patients with persistent symptoms, despite optimized medical therapy, is not clear. The open Nissen fundoplication has been associated with several complications in neurologically impaired children. In addition, postoperative morbidity rates of up to 50%, reoperation rates up to 20%, and mortality up to 50% have been reported.[39,40] More recently, the laparoscopic approach to the Nissen fundoplication has become the procedure of choice in the surgical management of GERD in general, and its results also appear superior among brain damaged children. Thus, Esposito and colleagues reported a 30% rate of postoperative complications and a 6% rate of reoperation.[41]

Swallowing disorders represent another common problem in this patient group, an occurrence that may further exacerbate GERD and esophagitis. Our group reported an incidence of 85.7% of swallowing disorders in patients with cerebral palsy.[33] Most patients showed dysfunction of the oral phase of swallowing, with abnormal formation of the food bolus due to either uncoordinated movements or contraction and rigidity of the tongue. Others, though demonstrating normal bolus formation, had huge defects in bolus propulsion toward the oropharynx, due to the lack of finely coordinated movements of the tongue against the palate. Swallowing disorders have significant implications for development, nutrition, respiratory health, and GI function in this group of patients.[33] The development of dysphagia is associated with a progressive reduction in food intake and it represents the main pathogenetic factor for malnutrition.[42] At the same time, swallowing disorders can cause recurrent episodes of pulmonary aspiration. Early diagnosis should be considered mandatory. A videofluoroscopic swallow study, being capable of simultaneously assessing pharyngeal motility and airways protection during the swallow, is considered the gold standard in children with neurologic impairment. Considering all of the problems related to oral feeding in these patients, a gastrostomy tube feeding is strongly recommended in neurologically impaired patients with dysphagia, undernutrition and associated respiratory diseases.[43–45] The American Academy of Cerebral Palsy and Developmental Medicine considers gastrostomy feeding as a valuable alternative nutritional source in this group of children, capable of improving nutrition, ameliorating GERD and associated pulmonary problems.[44]

Chronic Constipation

The prevalence of the chronic constipation varies from 25% to 75% among patients with cerebral palsy.[33] It represents a common but often underdiagnosed condition in patients with neurologic impairment. Chronic constipation is the result of prolonged colonic transit, which is secondary to an underlying gut dysmotility. In a study conducted by our group in 1994, colonic transit time seemed to be delayed predominantly in the left colon and rectum. These findings differentiate this form of constipation from that observed in patients with functional fecal retention.[46] In addition, we observed that, in contrast to neurologically normal children, none of the children with cerebral palsy presenting with chronic constipation reported fecal soiling.[33] Disruption of the neural modulation of colonic motility may play a predominant role in the development of constipation in neurologic disease. This could be a possible explanation for the poor impact of prokinetic drugs on delayed colonic transit in children with brain damage. A low fiber and fluid intake, as well as the frequent delay in diagnosis, certainly contribute to the development and reinforcement of constipation in neurologically impaired children. Our group demonstrated the efficacy of the dietary fiber glucomannan in improving bowel frequency in children with severe brain damage, despite no measurable effects on delayed transit.[47]

FAMILIAL DYSAUTONOMIA

Familial dysautonomia (FD), originally termed the Riley–Day syndrome, is an autosomal recessive disorder, occurring predominantly in the Ashkenazi Jewish population, with an incidence of about 1 in 1370 individuals. It is associated with a complex neurologic disorder that affects the sensory system and autonomic nervous system function.[48] The genetic defect affects prenatal neuronal development so that symptoms are present from birth. Although FD is caused by one gene and the penetrance is always complete, there is a great deal of variation in expression. The sensory dysfunction is characterized by alterations of small fiber neuronal populations such that FD patients have impaired sensations of temperature, pain, and vibration. The autonomic dysfunction affects multiple systems and is characterized by cyclic manifestations that feature the typical "dysautonomic crises"; these crises represent systemic reactions to physiologic and psychological stress: GI perturbations, such as vomiting, are a prominent component of the constellation of symptoms seen during an episode; other symptoms include hypertension, tachycardia, diaphoresis, personality changes, blotching of the skin, piloerection, functional ileus, and dilatation of the pupils.[49] Malfunction of the GI tract is the main clinical manifestation of FD, with impaired oropharyngeal coordination being one of the earliest symptoms. Uncoordinated swallowing is found in about the 60% of patients with FD and it is often responsible for the development of severe feeding problems, malnutrition, and recurrent aspiration, which can, in turn, lead to chronic lung disease. Cine-radiographic swallowing studies may help to document the degree of functional impairment and, accordingly, the extent to which normal swallowing function is retained.[50,51] According to Axelrod and colleagues, up to 80% of children will require a gastrostomy before their first birthday.[49] However, the prominent GI symptom is vomiting. Vomiting can occur cyclically as a part of dysautonomic crisis or daily in response to stress of arousal. The efficacy of diazepam in reducing vomiting during autonomic crisis suggests that the crisis is caused by a central phenomenon, probably arising from autonomic seizures.[52] GERD represents another frequent disorder in this special category of patients. Clinical symptoms can range from regurgitation, with obvious aspiration, to nocturnal episodes of wheezing, and apnea, to iron-deficiency anemia secondary to esophagitis. Sundaram and colleagues found a prevalence of 95% of GERD in a sample study of 174 FD patients.[53] A major contributor to the development of GERD is represented by dysfunction and increased relaxation of the lower esophageal sphincter.[54] The pathogenesis of GERD has been correlated to the degree of degeneration of the sympathetic nervous system and the consequent dominance of parasympathetic input. If an adequate and safe swallow is demonstrated and only GERD is identified, medical management, including thickening of feeds, positioning, and H2-antagonists, can be successfully tried. However, if symptoms persist and events such as hematemesis occur, fundoplication is usually performed combined with a gastrostomy.[55]

WILLIAMS SYNDROME

Williams syndrome (WS), also known as Williams–Beuren syndrome (WBS), is a multisystem disorder that occurs in 1/7500 births.[56] WS is due to a homozygous deletion of a contiguous gene at the long arm of chromosome 7 (7q11.23).[57] The majority of individuals with WS (99%) have a 1.5 megabase deletion in 7q11.23 encompassing the elastin gene (*ELN*) and 25 to 35 other genes, all of which are detectable by fluorescent in situ hybridization (FISH).[58] WS is characterized by dysmorphic facial features; mental retardation or learning difficulties; a unique cognitive profile; a distinctive personality; infantile hypercalcemia; and connective tissue abnormalities, including congenital heart defects, in particular supravalvular aortic stenosis.[59] GI symptoms such as chronic abdominal pain, feeding problems, constipation, and GERD are very common in children with WS. Constipation has been described in 40% of WS children.[60] Chronic abdominal pain is frequent in adolescents and may be related to constipation. However, complications such as hiatal hernia, peptic ulcer disease, cholelithiasis, diverticulitis, and ischemic bowel disease could also be responsible for the development of abdominal pain and have to be carefully excluded.[60] GERD may be present early in life and may be responsible for the development of esophagitis.[61] Hypercalcemia may exacerbate GI disorders, such as vomiting and constipation, and may cause irritability and muscle cramps; it is more common in infancy but may recur in adults.[62]

REFERENCES

1. Weijerman ME, de Winter JP. Clinical practice. The care of children with Down syndrome. Eur J Pediatr 2010;169:1445–52.

2. Spahis JK, Wilson GN. Down syndrome: perinatal complications and counseling experiences in 216 patients. Am J Med Genet 1999;89:96–9.
3. Moore SW. Down syndrome and the enteric nervous system. Pediatr Surg Int 2008;24:873–83.
4. van Trotsenburg AS, Heymans HS, Tijssen JG, et al. Comorbidity, hospitalization, and medication use and their influence on mental and motor development of young infants with Down syndrome. Pediatrics 2006;118:1633–9.
5. Carrascosa-Romero MC, Fernandez-Cordoba MS, Gonzalvez-Pinera J, et al. [Neurocristopathies: a high incidence of cerebral dysgenesis in patients with Hirschsprung's disease]. Rev Neurol 2007;45:707–12 [in Spanish].
6. Leffler A, Wedel T, Busch LC. Congenital colonic hypoganglionosis in murine trisomy 16—an animal model for Down's syndrome. Eur J Pediatr Surg 1999;9:381–8.
7. Nakazato Y, Landing BH. Reduced number of neurons in esophageal plexus ganglia in Down syndrome: additional evidence for reduced cell number as a basic feature of the disorder. Pediatr Pathol 1986;5:55–63.
8. Zarate N, Mearin F, Hidalgo A, et al. Prospective evaluation of esophageal motor dyfunction in Down's syndrome. Am J Gastroenterol 2001;96:1718–24.
9. Hillemeier C, Buchin PJ, Gryboski J. Esophageal dysfunction in Down's syndrome. JPGN 1982;1:101–4.
10. Weir K, McMahon S, Barry L, et al. Oropharyngeal aspiration and pneumonia in children. Pediatr Pulmonol 2007;42:1024–31.
11. Seki M, Kato T, Masutani S, et al. Pulmonary arterial hypertension associated with gastroesophageal reflux in a 2-month-old boy with Down syndrome. Circ J 2009; 73:2352–4.
12. Vandenplas Y, Rudolph CD, Di Lorenzo C, et al. North American Society for Pediatric Gastroenterology Hepatology and Nutrition, European Society for Pediatric Gastroenterology Hepatology and Nutrition. Pediatric gastroesophageal reflux clinical practice guidelines: joint recommendations of the North American Society for Pediatric Gastroenterology, Hepatology, and Nutrition (NASPGHAN) and the European Society for Pediatric Gastroenterology, Hepatology, and Nutrition (ESPGHAN). JPGN 2009; 49:498–547.
13. Bozinovski J, Poenaru D, Paterson W, et al. Esophageal aperistalsis following fundoplication in a patient with trisomy 21. Pediatr Surg Int 1999;15:510–1.
14. Wallace RA. Clinical audit of gastrointestinal conditions occurring among adults with Down syndrome attending a specialist clinic. J Intellect Dev Disabil 2007;32:45–50.
15. Okawada M, Okazaki T, Yamataka A, et al. Down's syndrome and esophageal achalasia: a rare but important clinical entity. Pediatr Surg Int 2005;21:997–1000.
16. Zarate N, Mearin F, Gil-Vernet JM, et al. Achalasia and Down's syndrome: coincidental association or something else? Am J Gastroenterol 1999;94:1674–7.
17. Azizkhan RG, Tapper D, Eraklis A. Achalasia in childhood: a 20-year experience. J Pediatr Surg 1980;15:452–6.
18. O'Kelly TJ, Davies JR, Tam PK, et al. Abnormalities of nitric-oxide-producing neurons in Hirschsprung's disease: morphology and implications. J Pediatr Surg 1994;29: 294–9.
19. Mearin F, Mourelle M, Guarner F, et al. Patients with achalasia lack nitric oxide synthase in the gastro-oesophageal junction. Eur J Clin Invest 1993;23:724–8.
20. Quinn FM, Surana R, Puri P. The influence of trisomy 21 on outcome in children with Hirschsprung's disease. J Pediatr Surg 1994;29:781–3.
21. Chakravarti A, Lyonnet S. Hirschsprung disease. In: Scrivner CR, Beaudet AR, Sly W, et al, editors. The metabolic and molecular bases of inherited disease. 8th edition. New York: McGraw-Hill; 2001. p. 6231–55.

22. Puffenberger E, Kauffman E, Bolk S, et al. Identity-by descent and association mapping of a recessive gene for Hirschsprung disease on human chromosome 13q22. Hum Mol Genet 1994;3:1217–25.
23. Arnold S, Pelet A, Amiel J, et al. Interaction between a Chromosome 10 RET Enhancer and Chromosome 21 in the Down Syndrome–Hirschsprung Disease Association. Hum Mutat 2009;30:771–5.
24. Zaahl MG, du Plessis L, Warnich L, et al. Significance of novel endothelin-B receptor gene polymorphisms in Hirschsprung's disease: predominance of a novel variant (561C/T) in patients with co-existing Down's syndrome. Mol Cell Probes 2003;17: 49–54.
25. Moore SW. The contribution of associated congenital anomalies in understanding Hirschsprung's disease. Pediatr Surg Int 2006;22:305–15.
26. Morabito A, Lall A, Gull S, et al. The impact of Down's syndrome on the immediate and long-term outcomes of children with Hirschsprung's disease. Pediatr Surg Int 2006; 22:179–81.
27. Wilson-Storey D, Scobie WG, Raeburn JA. Defective white blood cell function in Hirschsprung's disease: a possible predisposing factor to enterocolitis. J R Coll Surg Edinb. 1988;33:185–8.
28. Moore SW, Sidler D, Zaahl MG. The ITGB2 immunomodulatory gene (CD18), enterocolitis, and Hirschsprung's disease. J Pediatr Surg 2008;43:1439–44.
29. Catto-Smith AG, Trajanovska M, Taylor RG. Long-term continence in patients with Hirschsprung's disease and Down syndrome. J Gastroenterol Hepatol 2006;21: 748–53.
30. Kuban KC, Leviton A. Cerebral palsy. N Engl J Med 1994;330:188–95.
31. Staiano A, Cucchiara S, Del Giudice E, et al. Disorders of oesophageal motility in children with psychomotor retardation and gastro-oesophageal reflux. Eur J Pediatr 1991;150:638–41.
32. Wesley JR, Coran AG, Sarahan TM, et al. The need for evaluation of gastroesophageal reflux in brain-damaged children referred for feeding gastrostomy. J Pediatr Surg 1981; 16:866–71.
33. Del Giudice E, Staiano A, Capano G, et al. Gastrointestinal manifestations in children with cerebral palsy. Brain Dev 1999;21:307–11.
34. Hassal E, Kerr W, El-Serag HB. Characteristics of children receiving proton pump inhibitors continuously for up to 11 years duration. J Pediatr 2007;150:262–7.
35. Bohmer CJ, Klinkenberg-Knol EC, Niezen-de Boer RC, et al. The prevalence of gastro-oesophageal reflux disease based on non specific symptoms in institutionalized, intellectually disabled individuals. Eur J Gastroenterol Hepatol 1997;9:187–90.
36. Omari TI, Benninga MA, Sansom L, et al. Effect of baclofen on esophagogastric motility and gastroesophageal reflux disease. JPGN 2004;38:317–23.
37. Kawai M, Kawahara H, Hirayama S, et al. Effect of baclofen on emesis and 24-hour esophageal pH in neurologically impaired children with gastroesophageal reflux disease. JPGN 2004;38:317–23.
38. Miele E, Staiano A, Tozzi A, et al. Clinical response to amino acid-based formula in neurologically impaired children with refractory esophagitis. JPGN 2002;35:314–9.
39. Richards CA, Andrews PL, Spitz L, et al. Nissen fundoplication may induce gastric myoelectrical disturbance in children. J Pediatr Surg 1998;33:1801–5.
40. Richards CA, Carr D, Spitz L, et al. Nissen-type fundoplication and its effects on the emetic reflex and gastric motility in the ferret. Neurogastroenterol Motil 2000;12:65–74.

41. Esposito C, Van Der Zee DC, Settimi A, et al. Risks and benefits of surgical management of gastroesophageal reflux in neurologically impaired children. Surg Endosc 2003;17:708–10.
42. Campanozzi A, Capano G, Miele E, et al. Impact of malnutrition on gastrointestinal disorders and gross motor abilities in children with cerebral palsy. Brain Dev 2007; 29:25–9.
43. Schwarz SM, Corredor J, Fisher-Medina J, et al. Diagnosis and treatment of feeding disorders in children with developmental disabilities. Pediatrics 2001;108:671–6.
44. Samson-Fang L, Butler C, O'Donnell M; AACPDM. Effects of gastrostomy feeding in children with cerebral palsy: an AACPDM evidence report. Dev Med Child Neurol 2003;45:415–26.
45. Sullivan PB, Juszczak E, Bachlet AM, et al. Gastrostomy tube feeding in children with cerebral palsy: a prospective, longitudinal study. Dev Med Child Neurol 2005;47:77–85.
46. Staiano A, Del Giudice E. Colonic transit and anorectal manometry in children with severe brain damage. Pediatrics 1994;94(2 Pt 1):169–73.
47. Staiano A, Simeone D, Del Giudice E, et al. Effect of the dietary fiber glucomannan on chronic constipation in neurologically impaired children. J Pediatr 2000;136:41–5.
48. Axelrod FB. Familial dysautonomia. Muscle Nerve 2004;29:352–63.
49. Axelrod FB, Maayan C. Familial dysautonomia. In: Burg FD, Ingelfinger JR, Wald ER, Polin RA, editors. Gellis and Kagen's current pediatric therapy. 16th edition. Philadelphia: WB Saunders.
50. Krausz Y, Maayan C, Faber J, et al. Scintigraphic evaluation of esophageal transit and gastric emptying in familial dysautonomia. Eur J Radiol 1994;18:52–6.
51. Margulies SI, Brunt PW, Donner MW , et al. Familial dysautonomia. A cineradiographic study of the swallowing mechanism. Radiology 1968;90:107–12.
52. Axelrod FB, Zupanc M, Hilz MJ, et al. Ictal SPECT during autonomic crisis in familial dysautonomia. Neurology 2000;55:122–5.
53. Sundaram V, Axelrod FB. Gastroesophageal reflux in familial dysautonomia: correlation with crisis frequency and sensory dysfunction. JPGN 2005;40:429–33.
54. Linde LM, Westover JL. Esophageal and gastric abnormalities in dysautonomia. Pediatrics 1962;29:303–6.
55. Axelrod FB, Gouge TH, Ginsburg HB, et al. Fundoplication and gastrostomy in familial dysautonomia. J Pediatr 1991;118:388–94.
56. Stromme P, Bjornstad PG, Ramstad K. Prevalence estimation of Williams syndrome. J Child Neurol 2002;17:269–71.
57. Merla G, Ucla C, Guipponi M, et al. Identification of additional transcripts in the William's-Beuren syndrome critical region. Hum Genet 2002;110:429–38.
58. Lowery MC, Morris CA, Ewart A, et al. Strong correlation of elastin deletions, detected by FISH, with William's syndrome: evaluation of 235 patients. Am J Hum Genet 1995;57:49–53.
59. Greenberg F. Williams syndrome professional symposium. Am J Med Genet (Suppl) 1990;6:85–8.
60. Morris CA, Demsey SA, Leonard CO, et al. Natural history of Williams syndrome: physical characteristics. J Pediatr 1988;113:318–26.
61. de Montgolfier-Aubron I, Burglen L, Chavet MS, et al. [Early revealing of Williams-Beuren syndrome by digestive disorders]. Arch Pediatr 2000;7:1085–7 [in French].
62. Morris CA, Pober V, Wang P, et al. Medical guidelines for Williams syndrome. Available at: http://www.williams-syndrome.org/. Accessed September 13, 2011.

Paraneoplastic Gastrointestinal Dysmotility: When to Consider and How to Diagnose

John K. DiBaise, MD

KEYWORDS

- Paraneoplastic • Gastrointestinal • Motility disorder
- Cancer • Onconeural antibody

Gastrointestinal (GI) symptoms occur commonly in patients with cancer and may reflect dysfunction throughout the gut (**Box 1**). Many potential causes exist for these symptoms including GI dysmotility.[1] Although symptoms referable to disturbances in GI motor function are frequently encountered in patients with neoplasms, they are notoriously nonspecific and discrete disorders based on well-defined myoneural pathology are distinctly uncommon. Paraneoplastic neurologic syndromes are a heterogeneous group of rare disorders (**Box 2**) related to an underlying malignancy but caused by mechanisms other than metastases, metabolic and nutritional deficits, infections, ischemia, or side effects of cancer treatment.[2] A variety of antibodies directed against antigens expressed by both the tumor and the nervous system (ie, onconeural antibodies) has been reported in association with paraneoplastic syndromes helping to define different subtypes and, potentially, leading to an earlier diagnosis.[3] Recently, diagnostic criteria have been proposed to define a neurologic syndrome as paraneoplastic (**Box 3**).[4]

Although rare, there is a well-recognized association between malignant tumors and paraneoplastic GI dysmotility. While often affecting the entirety of the GI tract, paraneoplastic GI dysmotility may also affect isolated segments resulting in discrete syndromes (**Box 4**). In this review, paraneoplastic GI dysmotility will be discussed with an emphasis on when this entity should be considered in the differential diagnosis of GI dysmotility and how to confidently make the diagnosis.

The author has nothing to disclose.
Division of Gastroenterology and Hepatology, Mayo Clinic, 13400 East Shea Boulevard, Scottsdale, AZ 85259, USA
E-mail address: dibaise.john@mayo.edu

Gastroenterol Clin N Am 40 (2011) 777–786
doi:10.1016/j.gtc.2011.09.004
gastro.theclinics.com

Box 1
Gastrointestinal symptoms occurring in cancer patients

- Dysphagia
- Anorexia
- Early satiety
- Nausea
- Emesis
- Abdominal pain
- Constipation
- Diarrhea
- Fecal incontinence
- Weight loss

ETIOLOGY AND ANTIBODIES ASSOCIATED WITH PARANEOPLASTIC GI DYSMOTILITY

The etiology of paraneoplastic GI dysmotility appears to be immune-mediated – autoimmune, specifically. This is exemplified by the demonstration of onconeural antibodies (**Table 1**) selectively binding to enteric neurons in the myenteric plexus.[5–7] An autoimmune etiology of paraneoplastic GI dysmotility is also supported by the common presence of both concomitant paraneoplastic neurological syndromes that are also of suspected autoimmune origin and other autoantibodies (eg, parietal cell and thyroglobulin antibodies), rheumatoid factor, and circulating immune complexes in these patients.[8,9] An abnormality of external neural control by the autonomic nervous system has also been suggested.[10]

Paraneoplastic syndromes are characterized by an immune response to tumor antigens that are also present in nontumor cells. Apoptosis of tumor cells may expose

Box 2
Paraneoplastic neurologic syndromes

- Lambert-Eaton syndrome
- Limbic encephalitis
- Subacute cerebellar ataxia
- Sensory neuropathy
- Opsomyoclonus
- Encephalomyelitis
- Retinopathy
- Stiff-person syndrome
- Dermatomyositis
- Gastrointestinal dysmotility

Box 3
Diagnostic criteria for paraneoplastic neurologic syndromes

Definite

1. Classic syndrome and cancer develops within 5 years
2. Nonclassic syndrome but resolves/improves after cancer treatment without concomitant immunotherapy
3. Non-classic syndrome with associated onconeural antibodies and cancer develops within 5 years
4. Syndrome present with well-characterized onconeural antibodies and no cancer

Possible

1. Classic syndrome without onconeural antibodies and no cancer, but at high risk of underlying tumor
2. Syndrome present with partially characterized onconeural antibodies and no cancer
3. Nonclassic syndrome without onconeural antibodies and cancer develops within 2 years

Data from Graus F, Delattre JY, Antoine JC, et al. Recommended diagnostic criteria for paraneoplastic neurological syndromes. J Neurol Neurosurg Psychiatry 2004;75:338–40.

antigens which then stimulate antibody formation and activate cytotoxic T-cells. Immune destruction of the nontumor cells may then result in symptoms related to loss of normal function. In paraneoplastic GI dysmotility, presumably, tumor antigens elicit an immune response that cross-reacts with enteric or autonomic neural tissue leading to an immune attack directed against both the tumor and the respective nervous system.[11] Consistent with this hypothesis is a study in which mice injected systemically with IgG prepared from serum containing ganglionic-type acetylcholine receptors (AChRs) developed slowed GI transit, urinary retention, and other findings of dysautonomia.[12]

Paraneoplastic syndromes may affect any part of the central and peripheral nervous systems. Histologic abnormalities described in the myenteric plexus in the involved segment(s) of the gut that also support the autoimmune hypothesis include a decrease in the number of ganglion cells, replacement of neurons by Schwann cells and collagen, and a lymphoplasmacytic infiltrate.[13,14] Smooth muscle cells are typically unaffected. Recently, a loss of interstitial cells of Cajal was demonstrated in a patient with paraneoplastic dysmotility, suggesting that enteric neurons are not the only enteric target of paraneoplastic autoimmunity.[15] Despite these histologic

Box 4
Paraneoplastic GI dysmotility syndromes

- Achalasia and other types of esophageal dysmotility
- Gastroparesis
- Intestinal dysmotility including chronic intestinal pseudo-obstruction
- Constipation with or without megacolon
- Pelvic floor dyssynergia

Table 1
Onconeural antibodies associated with paraneoplastic GI dysmotility

Antibody	Tumor Types
ANNA-1	SCLC and thymoma
ANNA-2	SCLC and breast
VGCC, N-type	SCLC, non-SCLC, other carcinomas
VGCC, P/Q-type	SCLC, non-SCLC, other carcinomas
VGKC	SCLC, non-SCLC, other carcinomas
CRMP-5-IgG	SCLC, non-SCLC, other carcinomas
Ganglionic AChR	SCLC, non-SCLC, other carcinomas
Muscle AChR	SCLC, non-SCLC, other carcinomas
Striational	SCLC, non-SCLC, other carcinomas
PCA-1	Ovary and breast

AChR, acetylcholine receptor; ANNA, anti–neuronal nuclear antibody; CRMP, collapsing response-mediator protein; PCA, Purkinje cell cytoplasmic antibody; VGCC, voltage-gated calcium channel; VGKC, voltage-gated potassium channel.

findings and the presence of autoantibodies, the exact role of the antibodies in the pathogenesis of the organ dysfunction remains unclear. It has not been consistently demonstrated, for example, that the onconeural antibodies are themselves pathogenic for neurons, thus leading to the suggestion that these antibodies merely serve as markers of autoimmunity but do not participate in disease pathogenesis. Furthermore, the histologic nature of the underlying malignancy does not always dictate a certain autoantibody formation or specific dysmotility syndrome.[16]

The first and most common autoantibody recognized to be associated with paraneoplastic GI dysmotility is the type 1 anti–neuronal nuclear antibody (ANNA-1) also known as anti-Hu antibody. ANNA-1 recognizes the family of RNA nuclear binding proteins, Hu. These proteins are expressed in the neurons of the central, peripheral, and enteric nervous systems and are most commonly expressed in small cell lung cancer (SCLC)[17] but may also be expressed in multiple other tumor types.[18] Approximately 30% of patients with ANNA-1 autoimmunity have symptoms of GI dysmotility. The presence of ANNA-1 in the serum of SCLC patients has been shown to correlate with limited stage disease, response to chemotherapy, and improved patient survival, further supporting the autoimmune theory.[19] ANNA-2 (anti-Ri) antibodies also exist and have been associated with breast cancer and SCLC but, to date, have not been associated with paraneoplastic GI dysmotility.

The second most commonly reported antibodies in patients with paraneoplastic GI dysmotility target voltage-activated calcium channels. Calcium channels are classified as L, N, P/Q, R, and T channels. P/Q and N type channels are expressed in SCLC and are common targets of autoantibodies in such patients. They regulate acetylcholine release and participate in central and peripheral neurotransmission. Although these antibodies are reported more commonly with other paraneoplastic neurologic syndromes (eg, Lambert-Eaton syndrome), when associated with GI dysmotility, a search for an occult malignancy should be pursued.[20] The N type channel has also been associated with SCLC and retroperitoneal lymphomas.[21] These antibodies may coexist with ANNA-1 but have a weaker association with the eventual finding of a malignancy.

Antibodies directed against neuronal nicotinic acetylcholine receptors are also associated with both idiopathic and paraneoplastic forms of GI dysmotility.[22]

Antibodies targeting this protein can disrupt cholinergic synaptic transmission leading to autonomic failure. These antibodies appear to be directly pathogenic as their levels correspond to the severity of the autonomic failure and decrease with clinical improvement.[23]

Purkinje cell cytoplasmic autoantibody, type 1 (PCA-1, aka anti-Yo) targets a neuronal signal transduction protein Cdr. Although defined originally as a marker of paraneoplastic cerebellar degeneration, paraneoplastic GI dysmotility has been present in a small portion of PCA-1 seropositive patients in association with ovarian and breast cancer.[21] Other PCA autoantibodies include PCA-2 and PCA-Tr, which have been associated with SCLC and Hodgkin's lymphoma, respectively.

Other autoantibodies associated with SCLC include amphiphysin antibody and collapsing response-mediator protein 5 (CRMP-5) antibody. Approximately 20% of patients with the neuronal and glial cytoplasmic autoantibody, CRMP-5, have symptoms of GI dysmotility.[24]

CLINICAL PRESENTATION OF PARANEOPLASTIC GI DYSMOTILITY

Paraneoplastic GI dysmotility has been most commonly seen in association with SCLC, particularly in association with ANNA-1 positivity, but has also been described in relation to tumors of the stomach, esophagus, pancreas, breast, and ovary as well as ganglioneuroblastoma, bronchial carcinoid, retroperitoneal leiomyosarcoma, melanoma, and lymphoma, among others. A synchronous secondary malignancy has been described to occur in up to 13% of ANNA-1 positive SCLC patients.[18] Although active malignancy is usually present at the time of diagnosis of the paraneoplastic GI dysmotility, cases of paraneoplastic motility occurring in patients with a remote history of cancer currently in remission have also been reported.[8]

Paraneoplastic GI dysmotility is often rapidly progressive, leaving the affected patients debilitated in a matter of months. Indeed, a subacute (ie, less than 6 months) progressive clinical course and associated severe disability are highly suggestive of a paraneoplastic etiology to the GI dysmotility.[8,18,21] Nevertheless, a slowly progressive course, a relapsing course, or even a benign course does not reliably exclude the diagnosis. Given the rarity of these syndromes, little is known about their overall epidemiology, including gender distribution and age of onset. Some reports suggest that women are more likely to be affected, with a mean age of onset of 66 years.[8,25] However, a paraneoplastic cause should be considered, particularly in older men, given the generally higher prevalence of motility disorders in younger women. Although patients with paraneoplastic GI dysmotility may present with a dominant symptom suggesting isolated segmental GI involvement, most will have involvement of the entire gut and present with a wide variety of symptoms. In up to 80% of patients these symptoms may precede the diagnosis of the underlying tumor by weeks to years (usually within 6 months); occasionally, the tumor may only be diagnosed at autopsy. Indeed, in one of the larger case series, the GI dysmotility was observed to precede the diagnosis of SCLC by a mean of 8.7 months.[21] Many of these patients also have other neurologic, psychiatric, or chronic pain diagnoses and autoimmune disorders.[8] The main paraneoplastic GI dysmotility syndromes (see **Table 1**) will be briefly described next.

Dysphagia has been described with manometric and barium contrast study findings consistent with achalasia, and diffuse esophageal spasm has also been reported.[25,26] More common, however, are nonspecific peristaltic abnormalities.[21] Although most cases of pseudoachalasia do not reflect true paraneoplastic dysmotility, a small proportion of these patients have been shown to have no direct tumor involvement of the esophagogastric junction, often with ANNA-1 positivity.[26,27]

Gastroparesis is a commonly reported paraneoplastic GI syndrome,[10,21,25,28] occurring in 89% of individuals based on gastric emptying scintigraphy.[21] Dilation of the stomach has been noted on radiographic imaging studies and on gross examination at autopsy. Peripheral neuropathy and autonomic dysfunction may accompany gastric involvement.[10] Gastroparesis has been reported to be the most common paraneoplastic GI syndrome associated with ANNA-1 positivity.[18]

Chronic intestinal pseudo-obstruction may be the most common mode of presentation of paraneoplastic dysmotility reported and is certainly the most dramatic. Paraneoplastic intestinal pseudo-obstruction was first suggested in 1975[29] and is most often reported in association with SCLC and thymoma. The presence of lymphoplasmacytic infiltration of the myenteric plexus and circulating ANNA-1 antibodies are also characteristic findings. Radiographic imaging studies have revealed dilated small bowel and delayed transit through the small bowel. Gastroduodenal and small intestinal manometry studies have demonstrated findings consistent with neuropathy, such as absence of the phase III component of the migrating motor complex, postprandial antral hypomotility, lack of a fed pattern, and uncoordinated, prolonged bursts of phasic activity during both fasting and fed states.[6,21,30] Given the rarity of chronic intestinal pseudo-obstruction, a paraneoplastic cause should be considered in any patient who presents with typical features in association with undue weight loss and wasting, particularly when onconeural antibodies are present.

Constipation is a common symptom in paraneoplastic GI dysmotility; however, most will also demonstrate a dilated colon and/or evidence of a more diffuse pseudoobstruction syndrome.[10,21,25,29,31] An association with ganglionic acetylcholine receptor antibody has been reported in 2 patients with constipation and thymoma and SCLC.[23] Case reports have shown colonic dysmotility and severely slowed colonic transit and infiltration by T and B lymphocytes and plasma cells in the colonic myenteric plexus, in association with both ANNA-1 and antibodies against potassium channels.[31,32] Pelvic floor dyssynergia has also been reported in 4 patients, of whom 3had ganglionic AChR antibodies and 1 had coexisting voltage-gated potassium channel autoantibodies.[8] Formal evaluations of anorectal and colonic motility have not been performed.

DIAGNOSTIC APPROACH TO SUSPECTED PARANEOPLASTIC GI DYSMOTILITY

It is important to recognize that none of the syndromes listed in **Box 2** is exclusively paraneoplastic.[8] The incidence of malignancy in patients with suspected autoimmune GI dysmotility varies depending upon the symptoms and, in one report, ranged from 5% to 60%.[33] Unfortunately, other than an awareness that the clinical presentations of the paraneoplastic syndromes are often more severe than their nonparaneoplastic counterparts, there are no other clinical features that reliably differentiate paraneoplastic from nonparaneoplastic autoimmune GI dysmotility. In addition, despite the description of onconeural antibodies associated with many paraneoplastic syndromes, many of the antibodies may be found in different syndromes and a given syndrome may be associated with different antibodies. Furthermore, although the presence and type of onconeural antibody may define different subtypes of paraneoplastic syndromes, because less than 50% of patients with a paraneoplastic syndrome have onconeural antibodies,[4] the absence of these antibodies cannot exclude its diagnosis.

Although not specific for paraneoplastic GI dysmotility, gastrointestinal dysmotility should be confirmed by transit (eg, gastric emptying, colonic transit) and/or manometric (eg, esophageal, gastroduodenal, small bowel, colonic) testing depending up availability and presenting symptoms. At present, the detection of onconeural

Box 5
Factors that should raise the suspicion of paraneoplastic GI dysmotility

- Rapid symptom onset
- Significant weight loss
- History of smoking or other high cancer risk activity
- Strong family history of cancer
- Symptom onset later in life (? > 50–55 years of age), particularly in men
- Presence of concomitant autonomic or sensory neuropathy
- Presence of concomitant organ-specific autoantibodies*

*For example: glutamic acid decarboxylase (GAD) 65, islet cell antigen 512 (IA-2), gastric parietal cell, muscle striational, thyroid peroxidase, and thyroglobulin antibodies.

antibodies in a patient with suspected paraneoplastic GI dysmotility appears to be the most valuable diagnostic test.[21] These tests are available through commercial reference laboratories. There is insufficient evidence to support obtaining paraneoplastic antibodies in every patient with GI dysmotility; however, the presence of high risk or atypical features should prompt testing (**Box 5**).

The presence of gut dysmotility and positive ANNA-1 should prompt a search for an occult neoplasm, particularly SCLC. Even if the initial screen is negative (eg, CT imaging), a more aggressive search (eg, PET imaging, bronchoscopy, surgical exploration) should be considered and continued monitoring (eg, CT scanning at 6- to 12-month intervals) should be maintained in subsequent years given the lag period that is often present between the development of GI symptoms and the discovery of the malignancy.[18,21] Of note, reliance on plain films of the chest as the screening test of SCLC is not recommended given its demonstrated poor sensitivity (44% positivity in patients with proven SCLC and paraneoplastic GI dysmotility).[21] The presence of other antibodies, in the absence of ANNA-1, is less likely to predict the presence of malignancy. The value of full-thickness biopsy samples of the gut in diagnosis and in developing a treatment strategy remains unclear but may be of value in understanding the pathogenesis of these rare disorders. The risk of cancer detection/development decreases significantly 2 years after diagnosing a paraneoplastic neurologic syndrome and becomes very low after 4 years.

TREATMENT OF PARANEOPLASTIC GI DYSMOTILITY

The management of paraneoplastic syndromes, including paraneoplastic GI dysmotility syndromes, is generally centered on the treatment of the underlying malignancy. Indeed, to date, the best way to stabilize a paraneoplastic syndrome is to treat the tumor as soon as possible, further supporting the importance of early diagnosis.[34] Unfortunately, the prognosis is poor, with death often occurring within 12 months of the diagnosis. Although exceptions have been reported,[35,36] treatment of the underlying malignancy oftentimes does not lead to substantial improvement in the gut dysmotility even though the cancer may be put into remission.[10] Conventional measures used in the management GI dysmotility (eg, prokinetics, antiemetics, laxatives, and venting gastrostomy/enterostomy) and its complications (eg, small bowel bacterial overgrowth) appear to be of limited benefit. Management of the associated nutritional deficit with correction of micronutrient deficiencies and oral, enteral, or parenteral nutrition support, as needed, is important. With some exceptions,[8] aggressive immunosuppressive therapies such as high-dose corticosteroids, cyclophophamide, intravenous immunoglobulin, and plasmapheresis have been attempted without convincing success.[18,37] This may not be surprising given that, in the majority of paraneoplastic neurologic disorders, the symptoms are due to early and irreversible neuronal damage.[38]

SUMMARY

In this review of dysmotility in cancer patients, we have focused on paraneoplastic GI dysmotility as it provides an excellent example of how derangements of the neuromuscular apparatus of the gut can affect GI motility. A high index of clinical suspicion, together with serologic evaluation using a panel of autoantibodies in selected patients, is important in ensuring the early diagnosis of paraneoplastic GI dysmotility and may help guide management. Although it remains unproved that paraneoplastic antibodies are pathogenic, they are useful diagnostic markers. A better understanding of the pathogenesis of these disorders, including the role of paraneoplastic antibodies, will, hopefully, lead to earlier diagnosis and improved adjunctive, immunology-based treatments. Furthermore, even though successful treatment of the underlying cancer may not lead to reversal of the GI dysmotility, the recognition of a paraneoplastic syndrome may lead to early cancer diagnosis and a better chance of successful treatment of the cancer and overall survival. Although rare, it is imperative that clinicians be aware of the association between malignancy and GI dysmotility so that they know when to investigate for an underlying malignancy.

REFERENCES

1. DiBaise JK, Quigley EMM. Tumor-related dysmotility: gastrointestinal dysmotility syndromes associated with tumors. Dig Dis Sci 1998;4:1369–401.
2. Darnell RB, Posner JB. Paraneoplastic syndromes involving the nervous system. N Engl J Med 2003;349:1543–54.
3. Honnorat J, Antoine J-C. Paraneoplastic neurological syndromes. Orphanet J Rare Dis 2007;2:22.
4. Graus F, Delattre JY, Antoine JC, et al. Recommended diagnostic criteria for paraneoplastic neurological syndromes. J Neurol Neurosurg Psychiatry 2004;75:338–40.
5. Lennon VA, Sas DF, Busk MF, et al. Enteric neuronal antibodies in pseudoobstruction with small-cell lung cancer. Gastroenterology 1991;100:137–42.
6. Condom E, Vidal A, Rota R, et al. Paraneoplastic intestinal pseudo-obstruction associated with high titer of Hu autoantibodies. Virchows Arch Pathol Anat 1993;423: 507–11.
7. De Giorgio R, Bovara M, Barbara G, et al. Anti-HuD-induced neuronal apoptosis underlying paraneoplastic gut dysmotility. Gastroenterology 2003;125:70–9.
8. Dhamija R, Meng Tan K, Pittock SJ, et al. Serologic profiles aiding the diagnosis of autoimmune gastrointestinal dysmotility. Clin Gastroenterol Hepatol 2008;6:988–92.
9. Abu-Shakra M, Buskila D, Ehrenfeld M, et al. Cancer and autoimmunity: autoimmune and rheumatic features in patients with malignancies. Ann Rheum Dis 2001;60: 433–41.
10. Sodhi N, Camilleri M, Camoriano JK, et al. Autonomic function and motility in intestinal pseudoobstruction caused by paraneoplastic syndrome. Dig Dis Sci 1989;34:1937–42.
11. Maverakis E, Hoodarzi H, Wehrli LN, et al. The etiology of paraneoplastic autoimmunity. Clinic Rev Allerg Immunol 2011 Jan 19. [Epub ahead of print].

12. Vernino A, Ermilov LG, Sha L, et al. Passive transfer of autoimmune autonomic neuropathy to mice. J Neurosci 2004;24:7037–42.
13. Krishnamurthy S, Schuffler M. Pathology of neuromuscular disorders of the small intestine and colon. Gastroenterology 1987;93:610–39.
14. De Giorgio R, Guerrini S, Barbara G, et al. Inflammatory neuropathies of the enteric nervous system. Gastroenterology 2004;126:1872–83.
15. Pardi DS, Miller SM, Miller DL, et al. Paraneoplastic dysmotility: loss of interstitial cells of Cajal. Am J Gastroenterol 2002;97:1828–33.
16. Kashyap P, Farrugia G. Enteric autoantibodies and gut motility disorders. Gastroenterol Clin North Am 2008;37:397–410.
17. Kiers L, Altermatt HJ, Lennon VA. Paraneoplastic anti-neuronal nuclear IgG autoantibodies (type 1) localize antigen in small cell lung carcinoma. Mayo Clin Proc 1991;66:1209–16.
18. Lucchinetti CF, Kimmel DW, Lennon VA. Paraneoplastic and oncologic profiles of patients seropositive for type 1 antineuronal nuclear antibodies. Neurology 1998;50: 652–57.
19. Darnell RB, Posner JB. Paraneoplastic syndromes involving the nervous system. N Engl J Med 2003;349:1543–54.
20. Lennon VA, Kryzer TJ, Griesmann GE, et al. Calcium-channel antibodies in the Lambert-Eaton syndrome and other paraneoplastic syndromes. N Engl J Med 1995; 332:1467–74.
21. Lee HR, Lennon VA, Camilleri M, et al. Paraneoplastic gastrointestinal motor dysfunction: clinical and laboratory characteristics. Am J Gastroenterol 2001;96:373–9.
22. Vernino S, Adamski J, Kryzer J, et al. Neuronal nicotinic ACh receptor antibody in subacute autonomic neuropathy and cancer-related syndromes. Neurology 1998;50: 1806–13.
23. Vernino S, Low PA, Fealey RD, et al. Autoantibodies to ganglionic acetylcholine receptors in autoimmune autonomic neuropathies. N Engl J Med 2000;343:847–55.
24. Yu Z, Kryzer J, Griesmann GE, et al. CRMP-5 neuronal autoantibody: marker of lung cancer and thymoma-related autoimmunity. Ann Neurol 2001;49:146–54.
25. Chinn JS, Schuffler MD. Paraneoplastic visceral neuropathy as a cause of severe gastrointestinal motor dysfunction. Gastroenterology 1988;95:1279–85.
26. Liu W, Gackler W, Rice TW, et al. The pathogenesis of pseudoachalasia: a clinicopathologic study of 13 cases of a rare entity. Am J Surg Pathol 2002;26:784–8.
27. Gockel I, Eckardt VF, Schmitt T, et al. Pseudoachalasia: a case series and analysis of the literature. Scand J Gastroenterol 2005;40:378–85.
28. Berghmans T, Musch W, Brenez D, et al. Paraneoplastic gastroparesis. Rev Med Brux 1993;14:275–8.
29. Ahmed MN, Carpenter S. Autonomic neuropathy and carcinoma of the lung. Can Med Assoc J 1975;113:410–2.
30. Schuffler MD, Baird W, Fleming R, et al. Intestinal pseudo-obstruction as the presenting manifestation of small-cell carcinoma of the lung. A paraneoplastic neuropathy of the gastrointestinal tract. Ann Intern Med 1983;98:129–34.
31. Jun S, Dimyan M, Jones KD, et al. Obstipation as a paraneoplastic presentation of small cell lung cancer: case report and literature review. Neurogastroenterol Motil 2005;17:16–22.
32. Viallard JF, Vincent A, Moreau JF, et al. Thymoma-associated neuromyotonia with antibodies against voltage-gated potassium channels presenting as chronic intestinal pseudo-obstruction. Eur Neurol 2005;53:60–3.
33. Posner JB. Neurologic complications of cancer. Philadelphia: F.A. Davis; 1995.

34. Keime-Guibert F, Graus F, FLeury A, et al. Treatment of paraneoplastic neurological syndromes with antineuronal antibodies (anti-Hu, anti-Yo) with a combination of immunoglobulins cyclophosphamide, and methylprednisolone. J Neurol Neurosurg Psychiatry 2000;68:479–82.
35. Lautenbach E, Lichtenstein GR. Retroperitoneal leiomyosarcoma and gastroparesis: a new association and review of the literature. Am J Gastroenterol 1995;90:1338–41.
36. Hejazi RA, Zhang D, McCallum RW. Gastroparesis, pseudoachalasia and impaired intestinal motility as paraneoplastic manifestations of small cell lung cancer. Am J Med Sci 2009;338:69–71.
37. Graus F, Vega F, Delattre JY, et al. Plasmapheresis and antineoplastic treatment in CNS paraneoplastic syndromes with antineuronal autoantibodies. Neurology 1992; 42:536–40.
38. Vernino S, O'Neill BP, Marks RS, et al. Immunomodulatory treatment trial for paraneoplastic neurological disorders. Neuro-oncol 2004;6:55–62.

Chronic Intestinal Pseudo-Obstruction: Clinical Features, Diagnosis, and Therapy

Roberto De Giorgio, MD, PhD[a,b,*],
Rosanna F. Cogliandro, MD, PhD[a,b], Giovanni Barbara, MD[a,b],
Roberto Corinaldesi, MD[a,b], Vincenzo Stanghellini, MD[a,b]

KEYWORDS

- Chronic intestinal pseudo-obstruction
- Diagnosis of severe gut dysmotility • Enteric neuropathies
- Enteric myopathies • Abdominal radiology
- Intestinal manometry

Functional gastrointestinal disorders range from highly prevalent, but generally benign conditions, eg, functional dyspepsia and irritable bowel syndrome, to rare and potentially life-threatening diseases, eg, intestinal pseudo-obstruction syndromes. The term "intestinal pseudo-obstruction" was introduced in the late 1950s by Dudley and Colleagues who reviewed their own series observed over the years of thirteen cases with intestinal obstruction unexplained by any mechanical cause (notably, some of them originally referred to as "spastic ileus").[1] Subsequently, the existence of intestinal pseudo-obstruction syndromes has been confirmed and extended by other Authors.[2–4] It is now established that pseudo-obstruction refers to a condition characterized by symptoms and signs (both clinical and radiologic) of intestinal obstruction, but without evidence of any lesion occluding the lumen of the gut (hence the prefix "pseudo"). From a clinical standpoint, pseudo-obstruction syndromes may manifest either acutely or chronically.[5,6]

Acute intestinal pseudo-obstruction occurs in the vast majority of patients undergoing abdominal surgery (ie, postoperative ileus) and resolves spontaneously within a few days. It may also be caused by a number of conditions, such as peritonitis,

This work was supported by grants PRIN/COFIN from the Italian Ministry of University, Research and Education 2008 and 2010 (to R.DeG., G.B., and V.S.) and R.F.O. funds from the University of Bologna (R.DeG., G.B., R.C. and V.S.). R. De G. is the recipient of research grants from Fondazione Del Monte di Bologna e Ravenna.
The authors have nothing to disclose.
[a] Department of Clinical Medicine, University of Bologna, Italy Via Massarenti, 9, Building No. 5 (Nuove Patologie), St. Orsola-Malpighi Hospital, I-40138 Bologna, Italy
[b] Neurogastrenterology and Motility Laboratory, University of Bologna, Bologna, Italy
* Corresponding author.
E-mail address: roberto.degiorgio@unibo.it

Gastroenterol Clin N Am 40 (2011) 787–807
doi:10.1016/j.gtc.2011.09.005

hypokalemia, and myocardial infarction.[5,6] Acute colonic pseudo-obstruction (also referred to as Ogilvie's syndrome) belongs to these forms and is characterized by a massive colonic dilatation mainly affecting elderly people with underlying co-morbidities (eg, neurologic diseases, spinal or pelvic traumas).[7]

Like chronic heart failure, chronic intestinal pseudo-obstruction (CIPO) can be viewed as an insufficiency of the "intestinal pump" with defective smooth muscle contractility unable to promote transit of luminal contents through the gut, due to lack of either coordination or propulsive forces. The resulting clinical picture is characterized by recurrent episodes of intestinal subocclusion, basically undistinguishable from true mechanical obstruction.[8–10] This makes CIPO a clinical challenge often remaining undiagnosed or misdiagnosed for long periods.[8–10] In addition to severe dysmotility and related symptoms, CIPO is also a common cause of functional intestinal failure, being responsible for up to 20% of adult cases.[9,10] The reduction of the enteric absorptive surface below the minimal amount necessary for adequate digestion of nutrients makes nutritional supplementation a fundamental therapeutic measure in most patients with CIPO. The severity of the clinical picture, very often associated with disabling digestive symptoms between subocclusive episodes, together with the inability to maintain a normal body weight and the generally limited understanding of the syndrome by physicians are all factors contributing to poor quality of life and an established mortality rate in CIPO.[5–10]

This article will focus on practical issues that remain a matter of debate, such as histopathologic and pathogenetic data, clinical features, diagnosis, as well as main therapeutic measures currently available for adult patients with CIPO.

EPIDEMIOLOGY

CIPO is a typical example of a rare (or orphan) disease/syndrome with an unknown prevalence and incidence. Information derived from pediatric CIPO estimates that approximately 100 infants are born each year in the United States with congenital forms of CIPO,[6] which is undoubtedly an underestimate of the number of new cases per year. Overall, females appear more prone to CIPO than males as shown in major published series of adult patients.[9,11,12] Hopefully, registries developed by national health agencies will delineate the epidemiology of this syndrome based on accurate diagnosis in dedicated tertiary referral centers.

ETIOLOGY AND PATHOGENETIC FACTORS

Abnormalities of the gastrointestinal control systems, ie, smooth muscle cells, interstitial cells of Cajal (ICCs) as well as intrinsic and extrinsic nerves, can contribute to the severe motor derangement observed in patients with CIPO.[13,14] Neuro-ICC-muscular abnormalities in CIPO may be either secondary to a number of recognized diseases,[5,6,10,14] or idiopathic[5,8,9,10,13] when no accompanying disorders can be demonstrated. Furthermore, some cases of CIPO show a syndromic manifestation (ie, multisystem involvement) and familial clustering, thus suggesting a genetic origin.

In order to better understand the clinical management of CIPO, the next paragraphs will update the reader on the different forms and putative pathogenetic mechanisms of this challenging syndrome.

Secondary CIPO

Approximately half of the cases of CIPO are secondary to a wide array of diseases including neurologic, metabolic/endocrine, paraneoplastic, autoimmune, and infectious

Box 1
Main causes of secondary CIPO and related gut control system impairment

- *Extrinsic (sympathetic/parasympathetic) nervous systems*:

Stroke, encephalitis, calcification of basal ganglia, orthostatic hypotension, diabetes

- *Intrinsic (enteric) nervous system*

Paraneoplastic, viral infections, iatrogenic (anthraquinones), diabetes, Hirschsprung's disease, Chagas' disease, Von Recklinghausen's disease

- *Gastrointestinal smooth musculature (circular and longitudinal coats)*

Myotonic dystrophy, progressive systemic sclerosis

- *Mixed enteric nervous system and smooth muscle layer*

Scleroderma, dermatomyositis, amyloidosis, Ehlers-Danlos syndrome, jejunal diverticulosis, radiation enteritis

- *Undetermined*

Hypothyroidism, hypoparathyroidism, pheochromocytoma, iatrogenic (eg, clonidine, phenothiazines, antidepressants, antiparkinsonians, antineoplastics, bronchodilators)

diseases, which may impact at any number of levels on the enteric neuromuscular compartment and/or extraenteric organs with consequences on gut function (**Box 1**).[5,6,10] For example, several neurologic (eg, Parkinson's disease and Shy-Drager syndrome) and metabolic disorders (eg, diabetes mellitus) can affect the extrinsic (parasympathetic and/or sympathetic) nerve pathways supplying the digestive system. Paraneoplastic syndromes may evoke an inflammatory/immune infiltrate targeting neurons located in both submucosal and myenteric ganglia of the enteric nervous system (ENS); the cellular infiltrate along with circulating antineuronal antibodies are thought to damage the enteric reflexes thereby contributing to paraneoplastic dysmotility (see below). Many different neurotropic viruses may also cause morphologic (ie, inflammatory) or functional changes of the ENS and extrinsic neural pathways supplying the gut and are detectable in a subset of patients with CIPO.[15] Enteric smooth muscle cells can be selectively damaged in patients with myotonic dystrophy or progressive systemic sclerosis, while autoimmune disorders (eg, scleroderma, dermatomyositis and systemic lupus erythematosus), collagenopathies (eg, Ehlers-Danlos), jejunal diverticulosis and radiation enteritis can alter, not only enteric nerves, but also smooth muscle cells (and likely the ICC), resulting in a combined picture of neuro-myopathy.[5,6,10] Similar abnormalities to the neuro-ICC-muscular component are presumed to occur in rare cases of celiac disease associated with CIPO, as suggested by the presence of manometric abnormalities.[16] Other diseases such as hypothyroidism, hypoparathyroidism and pheochromocytoma are known causes of CIPO, although the type and degree of enteric neuro-ICC-muscular damage in these disorders is still a matter of investigation. Thus, because of this clinical heterogeneity, a comprehensive diagnostic work-up (see below) should always be performed in patients with CIPO in order to identify any possible underlying diseases and treat them accordingly.[10]

Genetic CIPO

Although most instances of CIPO are sporadic, different genetic forms have been reported.

Genes involved in the pathogenesis of congenital aganglionosis or Hirschsprung's disease, namely *GDNF* (glial-cell line derived neurotrophic factor), *GFRA1* (GDNF receptor-α_1), *EDN3* (endothelin 3), *EDNRB* (endothelin 3 receptor B), do not appear to play a role in autosomal dominant CIPO.[17] An exception to this is *SOX10*, a gene encoding for a transcription factor and *RET* regulator exerting an important role in neuronal survival and maintenance. Three sporadic patients carrying de novo *SOX10* heterozygous mutations showed a clinical phenotype of CIPO combined with some features of Waardenburg-Shah syndrome (ie, pigmentary anomalies and sensorineural deafness). In these patients full-thickness biopsy obtained at laparotomy revealed apparently normal ganglionic cells ruling out the diagnosis of Hirschsprung's disease.[18,19] Therefore, in addition to Hirschsprung's disease, *SOX10* abnormalities may contribute to a more diffuse derangement of gut dysmotility, such as CIPO.

Concerning autosomal recessive CIPO, a large Turkish consanguineous family with several members affected by severe dysmotility and recurrent subocclusive episodes, long-segment Barrett's esophagus and cardiac involvement was originally reported in 2003.[20] Homozygosity mapping has identified the locus on the region 8q23-q24,[21] although the specific gene responsible for this syndromic CIPO is still under investigation in our group. Another known form of recessive CIPO is the mitochondrial neurogastrointestinal encephalopathy (MNGIE).[22] In addition to severe gut dysmotility, patients with MNGIE manifest with cachexia, ptosis, ophthalmoparesis, peripheral neuropathy and exhibit white matter changes (leukoencephalopathy) on magnetic resonance imaging of the brain. This syndrome is caused by mutations in the thymidine phosphorylase gene (*TYMP*, also known as endothelial cell growth factor-1, *ECGF1*) or in the polymerase-γ gene (*POLG*, a form of MNGIE without leukoencephalopathy).[23,24] Gut tissue analysis showed that CIPO in patients with MNGIE is related to an underlying enteric myopathy.[25]

Two types of X-linked CIPO related to mutations of filamin A (*FLNA*) and L1 cell adhesion molecule (*L1CAM*) genes, both mapping on chromosome Xq28, have been reported. An *FLNA* mutation has been identified in a family with X-linked recessive CIPO with signs of central nervous system involvement.[26] In the other 2 families, where a duplication of the *FLNA* gene has been identified, CIPO was combined with patent *ductus arteriosus* and giant-platelet thrombocytopenia.[27] A recent histopathologic characterization of gut tissue specimens from five patients with FLNA mutations showed that myopathy, rather than neuropathy, accounts for the severe dysmotility of this familial form of CIPO.[28]

Finally, CIPO has been reported in patients with inherited degenerative smooth muscle and enteric neuronal disorders, termed familial visceral myopathy and neuropathy, respectively, but the underlying genes responsible for both clinical phenotypes have not been identified.

Histopathologic Features and Putative Mechanisms in CIPO

The majority of sporadic cases of CIPO has an undefined etio-pathogenesis. Nonetheless, the potential to collect full-thickness specimens via minimally invasive approaches and advances in the major techniques used to study biopsies (for further details see article by Knowles and Martin elsewhere in this issue) helped to minimize the uncertainty linked to previously labeled "idiopathic" CIPO.[14,29] Also, a better appraisal of the underlying neuro-ICC-muscular changes associated with CIPO and other gastrointestinal motility disorders has been recently proposed by the Gastro 2009 International Working Group on Gastrointestinal Neuromuscular Disorders (GINMD).[30] Accordingly, CIPO can be due to underlying neuropathies, myopathies and, although at a lower level of evidence, mesenchymopathies, based on neuronal, muscular or ICC involvement, respectively.[30] Nonetheless, it is worth noting that combined abnormalities, eg, neuro-myopathy, neuro-mesenchymopathy or other pictures, are increasingly recognized.[14,29,30]

There are 2 main histopathologic pictures of enteric neuropathies, namely inflammatory and degenerative.

Inflammatory (or immune-mediated) neuropathies are characterized by $CD3^+$ T lymphocytes (and, to a lower extent, plasma cells) infiltrating enteric neurons in the 2 ganglionated plexuses of the ENS (hence the term "enteric ganglionitis"). For still unclear reasons, the inflammatory infiltrate more commonly targets myenteric (ie, "myenteric ganglionitis") rather than submucosal ganglia. Also, axons giving off the myenteric ganglia and running throughout the muscular layer of the gut can exhibit an inflammatory axonopathy.[31]

Evidence of either enteric or myenteric lymphocytic ganglionitis in small bowel full thickness biopsies has been reported in 33 of 115 and in 17 of 50 patients with CIPO by Knowles and colleagues and Lindberg and colleagues, respectively.[32,33] Usually, the definition of lymphocytic ganglionitis is easily applicable when an overt infiltration of lymphocytes can be detected within myenteric ganglia.[31] However, a low-grade myenteric ganglionitis, characterized by a less prominent inflammatory cell infiltration, has been demonstrated in most CIPO and other forms of severe dysmotility.[32–34] Thus, a quantitative evaluation of the number of lymphocytes may be necessary for an appropriate diagnosis of an underlying inflammatory neuropathy. Although there are no normative data on the number of lymphocytes within myenteric ganglia in healthy controls, it has been proposed by the Gaströ 2009 International Working Group on GINMD that 5 or more lymphocytes per ganglion would be enough to indicate the presence of a myenteric ganglionitis.[35] Thus, Lindberg and colleagues found a low-grade ganglionitis in 59 patients with dysmotility (one-third of these had CIPO) and the mean number of lymphocytes/ganglion was 5.1.[33] Further research on lymphocytic ganglionitis will be necessary to establish the criteria for appropriate definition of this entity and actual pathogenetic relevance in CIPO. Lymphocytic myenteric ganglionitis may be associated with neuronal changes indicative of degeneration and loss up to complete ganglion cell depletion occurring in the most severe cases.[36]

Patients with lymphocytic myenteric ganglionitis may develop a humoral response characterized by antinuclear neuronal antibodies (ANNA-1 or, based on their molecular target, also referred to as anti-Hu).[37,38] These autoantibodies alter ascending reflex pathway of peristalsis in in vitro preparations, elicit neuronal hyperexcitability, evoke apoptotic and autophagic mechanisms in primary culture of myenteric neurons or neuronal cell lines.[38] Taken together, the lymphocytic infiltrate in myenteric ganglia and anti-neuronal autoantibodies can exert a pathogenetic role in patients with CIPO related to an inflammatory neuropathy.[39]

Other types of inflammatory neuropathies reported in CIPO are characterized by either eosinophils[40] or mast cells[41] infiltrating and/or surrounding myenteric ganglia. Given the limited number of patients so far reported, the clinicopathologic features of these peculiar forms of nonlymphocytic ganglionitis remain largely unclear.

Compared to inflammatory neuropathies, degenerative (noninflammatory) neuropathies are less well understood. Histopathologic findings may include a number of changes, ie, reduction of intramural (mainly myenteric) neurons associated with swollen cell bodies and processes, fragmentation and loss of axons.[29,35] Similar to neurodegenerative disorders of the central nervous system, mechanisms such as altered calcium signaling, mitochondrial dysfunction, and production of free radicals are thought to contribute to enteric neurodegeneration and loss.[29,35] Accordingly, apoptosis may also occur in the ENS of CIPO patients.[29,39] Few studies have accurately documented the prevalence of degenerative neuropathy in CIPO.[32,33,42] In our experience, ENS abnormalities characterized by frank degeneration were detected in 10 of 11 CIPO patients who had available histopathology.[9] Finally, glial cells, which exerts a key role in ENS maintenance and survival, can exhibit abnormalities (now referred to as gliopathy), which can account for enteric neuronal degeneration.[43] Although plausible, the existence of a gliopathy in CIPO needs to be confirmed.

As for neuropathies, enteric myopathies can also be categorized into inflammatory and degenerative forms. Inflammatory myopathies, also referred to as leiomyositis, are characterized by an immune infiltrate, mainly composed by $CD4^+$ and $CD8^+$ lymphocytes; thus they can be considered the muscular counterpart of inflammatory neuropathies. Adult cases of leyomiositis with an associated clinical picture of severe CIPO have been reported.[44,45] If not arrested by immunosuppressive therapy (see later), the progression of leiomyositis may be life-threatening as it evolves toward major disruption of both circular and longitudinal muscle coats throughout the gut.[45]

Regarding degenerative myopathies, both familial and sporadic forms have been recognized. The histopathologic features do not permit differentiation between sporadic and familial myopathies as smooth muscle cell vacuolization and fibrosis can be detected in both. Familial visceral myopathy (FVM, also referred to as "hollow visceral myopathy")[46] encompasses at least 2 phenotypes, namely type I and II. FVM type I is autosomal dominant and associated with gastrointestinal (megaesophagus, megaduodenum) and extragastrointestinal (megacystis, mydriasis) manifestations.[47] FVM type II is autosomal recessive and corresponds to MNGIE. Vacuolization and fibrosis are mainly localized to the longitudinal, rather than circular, muscle layer of the small bowel with the resultant formation of diverticula.[22,25] In sporadic degenerative myopathy, smooth muscle vacuolization and fibrosis affect both circular and longitudinal layers of the intestinal wall.[14,30,35] The prevalence of myopathy in CIPO has been shown to be quite low in most reported series,[32,33] with the exception of one study by Mann and colleagues who found more myopathic than neuropathic CIPO.[42] None of our 11 cases of CIPO had signs indicative of smooth muscle damage.[9] In order to improve the diagnostic yield of gut muscle pathology, Wedel and colleagues investigated different specimens from patients with severe dysmotility, including slow transit constipation, idiopathic megacolon, Hirschsprung's disease, but not cases of CIPO, using immunohistochemical analysis with a panel of different smooth muscle markers (ie, smooth muscle myosin heavy chain [SMMHC], smoothelin [SM] and histone deacetylase 8 [HDAC8]).[48] Compared to classic histochemical techniques (H&E, Masson's trichrome) and smooth muscle alpha-actin (alpha-SMA) immunolabeling, which turned out to be normal, the expression of SMMHC, SM and HDAC8 was either absent or focally lacking in Hirschsprung's disease (80%), idiopathic megacolon (75%) and slow-transit constipation (70%). These findings, which have been confirmed by ultrastructural evaluation, indicate subtle (ie, molecular) changes otherwise undetectable with routine stains or alpha-SMA immunohistochemistry.[48] Similar changes to SMMHC, SM and HDAC8 immunolabeling may be expected to occur in CIPO, but supportive data are needed.

ICC network abnormalities (also labeled as mesenchymopathies) have been detected in patients with CIPO.[35,49] In our hands, decreased ICC density, loss of processes and damaged intracellular cytoskeleton and organelles, as revealed by c-Kit immunohistochemistry have been detected in 5/11 CIPO patients.[9] Given the significant physiologic role exerted by ICCs in gut motility, it has been proposed that their impairment may contribute to the enteric dysmotility leading to CIPO. Nonetheless, the International Working Group on gastrointestinal neuromuscular pathology

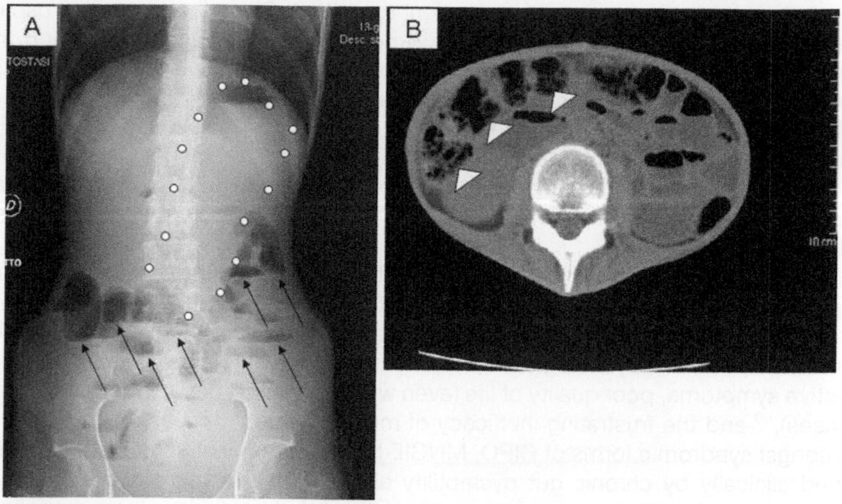

Fig. 1. Plain x-ray abdominal film of a 29-year-old female patient with idiopathic CIPO during an acute subocclusive episode. *(A)* Marked gastric distention (*encircled by white dots along the area occupied by the distended stomach*) and multiple air-fluid levels mainly of small bowel loops (*black arrows*). *(B)* High-resolution CT scan confirmed the marked gastrectasia and small bowel loop distention with abundant fluid contents (*white arrowheads*). The small bowel wall appeared normal, while the colon showed evidence of impacted stools (ie, coprostasis).

considered it as yet premature to attribute an etiologic role to ICC changes in several gut motility disorders, with the exception of diabetic gastroparesis.[30]

CLINICAL FEATURES

Although the small bowel is usually worst affected, CIPO may involve any segment of the gastrointestinal tract and patients present with clinical manifestations that may vary with the natural evolution of the disease over time.[5,10–14] In addition, extragastrointestinal manifestations and the degree of malnutrition also contribute to the clinical features of the syndrome.[5,10–14]

In general, the predominant symptoms reported by patients include abdominal pain/discomfort, sometimes localized to the periumbilical and epigastric region, but more frequently diffuse over the whole abdomen, along with bloating and distention. Sub-occlusive episodes are characterized by abrupt onset of intense, cramping pain, abdominal distention, nausea and vomiting. Plain radiograph of the abdomen during acute episodes demonstrates typical bowel loop distention and air-fluid levels in the upright position (**Fig. 1**A), providing a picture resembling mechanical obstruction; a key diagnostic feature. Because of suspected mechanical obstruction, patients may be often erroneously referred to surgery. Hence, a history of unnecessary, repeated exploratory laparotomy is a clinical hallmark of patients with CIPO. On the other hand, in most cases with a known history, conservative measures, ie, naso-gastric suction and fluid and electrolyte, resolve symptoms. After the acute episode, patients may became completely asymptomatic or, more often, continue to experience severe digestive symptoms suggestive of delayed transit in the proximal (eg, anorexia, early satiety nausea and vomiting) and/or distal (constipation) portions of the gut. The prevalence and severity of acute exacerbations, which recur at irregular intervals and without detectable triggers, vary from patient to patient. Since food ingestion usually worsens digestive symptoms, patients stop oral nutrition for long periods and this aggravates malnourishment related to dysmotility. Impaired intestinal transit with chronically dilated bowel loops is a major factor contributing to malabsorption, which is a further cause of weight loss. Also, because of intestinal stasis, up to 30% of CIPO patients may complain of diarrhea (or sometimes steatorrhea), almost invariably due to bacterial overgrowth.[9] Paradoxically, a deterioration in symptoms with reappearance of intractable constipation, may occur when antibiotics are used to treat bacterial overgrowth.

Gastroparesis and urinary bladder dysfunction (with or without megacystis and megaureter) can be frequently associated with neuropathic and, especially, myopathic CIPO and probably share common pathophysiologic mechanisms. Finally, depression or other psychological disorders may develop as a result of disabling digestive symptoms, poor quality of life (even worse than that of patients with organic diseases),[50] and the frustrating inefficacy of most therapeutic measures.[51]

Amongst syndromic forms of CIPO, MNGIE is one of the best characterized and is defined clinically by chronic gut dysmotility along with 2 or more of the following neurologic manifestations: progressive external ophthalmoplegia, ptosis, peripheral polyneuropathy, magnetic resonance imaging appearances consistent with cerebral leukoencephalopathy, and sensorineural hearing loss. A familial history, coupled with the absence of any other identifiable cause for chronic intestinal subocclusion may be a relevant clinical feature of MNGIE.[22,52]

Patients with secondary CIPO should be carefully examined for systemic manifestations suggestive of an underlying condition. Briefly, proximal muscle weakness may indicate polymyositis/dermatomyositis. Scleroderma is commonly associated with classic skin abnormalities, while paraneoplastic syndrome with involvement of central and/or enteric nervous system(s) should prompt investigation aimed to disclose an occult malignancy of the lung, breast, and ovary (the article by John K. DiBaise elsewhere in this issue). Hematologic tumors, eg, multiple myeloma or Hodgkin's lymphoma, should also be sought. CIPO related to Chagas' disease may be common in parts of Latin America and is characterized by concomitant dysphagia and cardiomyopathy.[5,6,10,31,36,38,39]

DIAGNOSIS

The diagnosis of CIPO is basically clinical and it is established when mechanical causes of gastrointestinal subocclusion have been carefully excluded. The main criteria to differentiate mechanical from "functional" subocclusion, either acute or chronic, have been summarized in **Table 1**. Also, the clinical manifestations and major associated conditions, which may lend a hand in the diagnosis of CIPO, have been listed in **Box 2**. A thorough diagnostic work-up is mandatory for 3 reasons: (a) to confirm the actual absence of mechanical obstruction of the gut; (b) to identify underlying diseases responsible for secondary forms of CIPO; and (c) to explore possible pathophysiologic features of idiopathic CIPO and possibly reveal complications. In achieving these ends, radiologic, endoscopic, laboratory, manometric, and, whenever clinically indicated, histopathologic studies may all play an important role.

Radiology

Radiology is fundamental for the diagnosis of CIPO as it identifies typical signs of intestinal occlusion (air-fluid levels on plain x-ray abdominal films) and excludes organic causes of mechanical obstruction (by contrast studies or computerized tomography). Air-fluid levels are best visualized with the patient in the upright position

Table 1
Main differences between mechanical *vs* functional intestinal obstruction

	Mechanical obstruction	POI	AIPO/ACPO	CIPO
Luminal obstruction	Yes	No	No	No
Motility	Initially ↑ then ↓ proximal to obstruction	↓	↓/uncoordinated	↓/uncoordinated
Dilatation	Yes (proximal to obstruction)	No	Yes	Yes
GI involvement	Proximal to obstruction	Mainly small bowel	Mainly colon	Pan-enteric
Radiology	Typical "cut-off" point; presence of air-fluid levels	"Cut-off point" occasionally present; air-fluid levels usually absent	"Cut-off point" occasionally present; air-fluid levels sometimes detected	"Cut-off point" occasionally present; air-fluid levels detectable
Course	Acute	Acute	Acute	Chronic
Progression	Rapidly evolving toward total obstruction	Self-limiting, slowly improving	May respond to medical treatment; major complication may occur	Variable, generally self-limiting
Treatment	Surgery	Supportive measures	Medical treatment (neostigmine); decompressive endoscopy or surgery in unresponsive cases	Variable; EN, TPN/HPN often needed

Abbreviations: ↑ = increased; ↓ = decreased; AIPO/ACPO, acute intestinal pseudo-obstruction/acute colonic pseudo-obstruction; CIPO, chronic intestinal pseudo-obstruction; EN, enteral nutrition; GI, gastrointestinal; POI, postoperative ileus; TPN/HPN, total/home parenteral nutrition.

Box 2
Clinical manifestations suggestive of CIPO

Principal clinical and radiologic features

- Repeated, inconclusive abdominal surgery
- Recurrent episodes of abdominal pain, distention and inability to defecate (± vomiting)
- Distended bowel loops and air-fluid levels in the upright position during acute episodes
- Lack of mechanical causes of gastrointestinal obstruction

Associated conditions/symptoms

- Esophageal motor disorders
- Gastroparesis
- Diarrhea/malabsorption (due to small intestinal bacterial overgrowth)
- Urinary tract dysfunction (megacystis, megaureter) and related symptoms
- Underlying diseases associated with secondary CIPO

Other findings

- Family history of similar digestive disorders
- Weight loss despite dietary modifications/supplementation
- Need for parenteral nutrition
- Visible movements of distended bowel loops through a thin abdominal wall
- Abnormal motor patterns at small bowel manometry

(see **Fig. 1**A) although this may be difficult to achieve during acute episodes. Contrast follow-through studies may disclose a marked intestinal distention (sometimes involving the stomach and duodenum) as well as uncommon findings, eg, small bowel diverticulosis (particularly in cases related to MNGIE), and pneumatosis intestinalis (ie, gas in the intestinal wall). However, the diagnostic validity of this technique is considerably hampered by flocculation of barium (or water-soluble) meal in distended bowel loops of patients with CIPO. Therefore, the contrast follow through examination has been largely superseded by computed tomography (CT), which accurately assesses the gut wall and identifies adhesions resulting from repeated laparotomies, and the new multidetector-row helical CT (MDCT),[53] which provides even more detailed and accurate information (see **Fig. 1**B). Excretory urograms should be performed in patients with urinary symptoms, since diffuse neuromyopathies may affect both gastrointestinal and urinary system. A chest CT may be necessary to exclude small-cell lung cancer in patients with suspected paraneoplastic syndrome (eg, middle-aged heavy smokers with rapidly progressive deterioration of the general conditions). Finally, brain imaging is required to identify leukoencephalopathy in cases of CIPO related to MNGIE.[25,52]

Endoscopy

Endoscopy can help to identify mechanical occlusions in the upper (gastrojejunal) and lower (ileocolonic) gut. Upper gastrointestinal endoscopy is useful to exclude an aortomesenteric artery compression syndrome, which may be difficult to differentiate on imaging from CIPO due to the impact of severe dysmotility on this segment of the small intestine (ie, sustained uncoordinated contractions in the distal duodenum).[8] The duodenal mucosa should be biopsied to exclude celiac disease. Future approaches, such as, natural orifice transluminal endoscopic surgery (NOTES),[54] will increase the diagnostic role of endoscopy in severe motility disorders by providing full thickness biopsy samples for histopathology.[54]

Laboratory Tests

Laboratory examinations can be useful to identify secondary forms of CIPO related to potentially curable diseases (see above). Thus, serum glucose, thyroid-stimulating hormone, complete blood count, albumin, liver enzymes, vitamin B12, inflammatory indexes (eg, C-reactive protein and erythrocyte sedimentation rate), and autoantibody profile should be all tested.[51] Identification of circulating antineuronal antibodies, such as ANNA-1/anti-Hu, should be sought in patients with paraneoplastic syndrome.[31,38] Patients on TPN or, who are, in general, unable to maintain oral feeding should be monitored for fluid and electrolyte balance and circulating levels of essential elements. Finally, patients with MNGIE should be tested for lactic acid (at rest and during exercise), thymidine phosphorylase levels in the buffy coat, nucleotide concentrations, and genetic analysis.[52]

Manometry

Although not available in most centers, the evaluation of the small bowel pressure profile by standard or ambulatory manometry may be an important adjunct in the diagnostic process of CIPO.[8–12] First, this technique may help in differentiating mechanical from functional forms of subocclusion, the former being characterized by postprandial, prolonged, high-pressure, nonpropagated contractions.[5,6,8,10] Second, gut manometry may provides some indication of the origin of the underlying dysmotility, that is, myogenic or neurogenic CIPO.[5,6,8,10] In neuropathic CIPO, contractions are uncoordinated although they have normal amplitude; conversely, in myopathic forms, intestinal contractions are coordinated but of low amplitude, when at all recordable by current manometric techniques. Nonetheless, low amplitude contractions may be due to the inability of the manometric catheter to record nonocclusive contractions as occurs when bowel loops are dilated. Altered neurogenic motor patterns include abnormal activity fronts, bursts of uncoordinated contractions, sustained uncoordinated contractions and the inability to respond to meal ingestion.[5,6,8,10] However, since similar abnormalities can be recorded in a variety of clinical conditions which are not characterized by subocclusive episodes, the diagnosis of CIPO can not be exclusively based on manometric findings.[55] Esophageal manometry is generally not useful unless patients have scleroderma-related CIPO. Anorectal manometry is indicated only if the clinical picture is characterized by intractable constipation and marked large bowel distention suggestive of Hirschsprung's disease.

Histopathology

An appropriate and well performed histopathologic analysis of full thickness biopsies from patients with CIPO may be diagnostic by disclosing the cellular abnormalities underlying gut dysmotility. Also important indicators relevant to the prognosis and management of patients with CIPO may be identified, such as detection of an underlying neuropathy, myopathy, or ICC abnormality, either alone or in combination. However, the enthusiasm for obtaining tissue for histopathology has been tempered by a number of factors including the common experience that surgery may worsen the underlying dysmotility and/or promote the formation of adhesions, which further complicate the clinical picture; discouraging pathologic reports describing an "apparently normal" neuromuscular layer even in cases featuring marked bowel loop distention and severe dysmotility; and, finally, the relatively scanty amount of normative data on the quantitative analysis of human gut neuromuscular tissues.[56] These and other issues have been partly overcome by some important advances: (1) the use of minimally invasive approaches (ie, laparoscopic surgery) for collecting full-thickness biopsy samples with a high diagnostic yield and safety[57] and (2) recently established guidelines defining technical characteristics and histopathologic reporting in GINMD.[35] Practical aspects, such as which gut segment should be biopsied, tissue collection and processing, and reporting of results and other aspects of GINMD, including CIPO, have been detailed by the Gastro 2009 International Working Group[35] (see article by Knowles and Martin elsewhere of this issue of *Gastroenterology Clinics of North America*). Future developments offer considerable promise and include the possibility of obtaining diagnostic information on the ENS from mucosal biopsies (eg, at colonoscopy) through an assessment of the submucosal plexus[58] as well as the use of new endoscopic techniques, eg, NOTES to obtain full-thickness biopsies.[54]

NATURAL HISTORY

Both pediatric and adult CIPO patients show an invariably severe clinical course **Table 2**.[9,11,12,42] Unfortunately, the lack of stringent diagnostic criteria to ensure the inclusion of homogeneous patient populations in long-term outcome studies limits the interpretability of such studies. In our experience, based on 59 adult patients with established idiopathic CIPO followed up for a long period of time (up to 13 years), the first subocclusive episode was often preceded by nonspecific, progressively severe digestive symptoms over a time-frame of 1 to 46 years.[9] An acute onset occurred in approximately 25% of the cases, while the median time between the first subocclusive episode and diagnosis was 8 years, with most patients (about 88%) undergoing about 3 worthless surgical procedures. Digestive symptoms worsened over time, with abdominal pain becoming intractable or responsive only to major analgesic drugs, ie, opioids, in about 20% to 25% of patients.[9,42] Most patients had restrictions to oral feeding, while 30% to 50% required long-term total or home parenteral nutrition (TPN/HPN).[9,12,42] Overall, all studies indicate a number of disease-related complications (eg, surgery, parenteral nutrition, transplantation and septic-shock) which account for high mortality rates (from about 10% up to 34%).[9,11,12,42] In the study by Amiot and colleagues, which was based on patients with CIPO who were all on HPN, a lower mortality was associated with the ability to restore oral feeding at baseline and symptom occurrence before the age of 20 years, while a higher mortality was associated with the presence of systemic sclerosis.[11] Two manometric parameters, an inadequate/absent motor response to meals and generalized hypomotility have been shown to be predictive of poor outcome in patients with CIPO.[9,12]

THERAPY

The objectives of the treatment of CIPO are 3-fold: (a) to maintain an adequate caloric intake, limit malnutrition and avoid dehydration; (b) to promote coordinated gastrointestinal motility; and (c) to treat complications (eg, bacterial overgrowth and intractable pain), or the underlying disease (in secondary forms of CIPO). In general, current therapeutic approaches are still far from effective for patients with CIPO; nonetheless, it should be recognized that recent refinements in nutritional,

Table 2
Summary of studies reporting the clinical outcome of adult patients with CIPO

Author Ref Patient Design Follow-up (months)	Outcome (no. of patients)
Mann and colleagues, 1997[42] 20 idiopathic CIPO Cross-sectional (unspecified)	Nutrition: normal (n = 8); enteral (n = 2); parenteral (n = 8) Opiate dependence (n = 5) Mortality (n = 2): myocardial infarction from extensive caval thrombosis in one case; bronchopneumonia in the other
Stanghellini and colleagues, 2005 [9] 59 idiopathic CIPO Prospective 55 (12-156) months	↓ frequency of subocclusive episodes (n = 41) Nutrition: inability to maintain oral feeding (n = 36); TPN/HPN (n = 16) Intractable pain (n = 12) Small bowel transplantation (n = 3) Mortality (n = 5): TNP-related complications in four patients; postintestinal transplant complications in one case
Amiot and colleagues, 2009 [11] 51 with both primary (n = 34) and secondary (n = 17) CIPO all in HPN Retrospective 8.3 (0-29) years	Surgical procedures (n = 43) leading to short-bowel syndrome in a subset of patients (n = 19) Nutrition: actuarial HPN dependence in 94, 75, and 72% at 1, 2, and 5 years, respectively Survival probability: 94, 78, 75, and 68% at 1, 5, 10, and 15 years Lower mortality: associated with restoration of oral feeding at baseline and symptom occurrence before the age of 20 years Higher mortality: associated with systemic sclerosis Intestinal transplantation in none
Lindberg and colleagues, 2009 [12] [55]with both primary and secondary CIPO Retrospective 9.9 (5.2-20.1) years	Nutrition: TPN/HPN (n = 27) Manometry: absence of fed motor response to meals (n = 16/43); severe hypomotility (n = 7) Mortality in n = 19 patients

Legend: ↓ = decreased; CIPO, chronic intestinal pseudo-obstruction; TPN/HPN, total/home parenteral nutrition.

Table 3
Therapeutic trials in adult patients with CIPO

Author Ref Patient Design Duration of study Treatment regimen	Effects
Camilleri and colleagues, 1989[60] 26 patients (15 with intestinal dysmotility or CIPO) Parallel groups 6 weeks Cisapride 10 mg t.i.d. vs. placebo	No significant differences of overall symptom response ↑ gastric emptying of solids
Abell and colleagues, 1991[61] 21 patients (12 with CIPO) Open trial 12 months Cisapride 10 mg t.i.d.	No significant differences on symptom response ↑ gastric emptying of solids
Soudah et al, 1991 [62] 5 patients with scleroderma-related CIPO + SIBO Open trial 3 weeks Octreotide 100 mcg s.c.	↓ bacterial overgrowth ↓ symptom score for nausea, vomiting, bloating and abdominal pain
Camilleri and colleagues, 1994[63] 37 neuropathic patients (gastroparesis or intestinal dysmotility or CIPO) Parallel groups 12 weeks Cisapride 10 and 20 mg t.i.d. vs. placebo	No significant effect of treatment on overall symptom score ↓ overall symptom score at 6 weeks and 12 weeks in patients without vagal dysfunction and in patients with generalized sympathetic dysfunction, respectively

Verne and colleagues, 1995[64] 14 patients with scleroderma-related CIPO Open trial 20-33 weeks Octreotide 50 mcg s.c. o.d. + erythromycin 200 t.i.d. orally	Long-term improvement of nausea and abdominal pain (n = 5)
Camilleri and colleagues, 1996[65] 37 patients with neuropathy (gastroparesis or intestinal dysmotility or CIPO) Open trial 12 months Cisapride 20 mg t.i.d.	Improvement of overall symptom score No significant change in body weight Improvement of overall symptom score in the presence of general sympathetic dysfunctions and in the absence of vagal dysfunctions
Emmanuel and colleagues, 2004[66] 15 patients with CIPO Open, retrospective responders to erythromycin (n = 6 patients) 41 months (13-64) Erythromycin 1.5-2.0 g/day i.v. or orally	↑ overall symptomatic score (n = 6) Improved vomiting (n = 5) ↑ body weight (n = 4)

Abbreviations: ↓ = decreased; ↑ = increased; CIPO, chronic intestinal pseudo-obstruction; i.v., intravenously; o.d., once/day; patients, patients; s.c., subcutaneously; SIBO, small intestine bacterial overgrowth; t.i.d, three times/day.

pharmacologic, and surgical options have helped to improve the management of the disease.[10,51]

Nutritional Support

Patients with CIPO are often malnourished, due to malabsorption and inadequate food intake related to severe digestive symptoms. Liquid or homogenized, hypocaloric, low fat and low residue meals may be indicated for patients with adequate intestinal absorption. Vitamin levels, especially vitamins A, D, E, and K, as well as B12 and folic acid, should be checked and, if necessary, supplemented. Enteral or parenteral nutrition should be considered for patients unable to maintain sufficient oral feeding. Enteral feeding is recommended in patients with upper (eg, stomach and duodenum) or more localized gastrointestinal tract impairment. The placement of feeding tubes above the level of the gut segments primarily affected by dysmotility will only serve to compromise the outcome of enteral nutrition and worsen digestive symptoms. As for parenteral, enteral nutrition should be started as a slow infusion over many hours during the day; a progressive increase in the volume and caloric content may be used as an indirect way of challenging the functional absorptive capacity of the gut. In the most severe cases, TPN is necessary to maintain nutritional support and adequate hydration.[59] The infusion velocity of nutrients should be set to keep patients free of infusion for some time during the day. This (with occasional intake of oral foods, if at all possible) may help to decrease the distress that is unavoidably associated with TPN. Complications of TPN, including liver insufficiency, pancreatitis, glomerulonephritis, and catheter-related thrombosis and septicemia, are frequent causes of death in any form of CIPO.[59] Finally, individualizing TPN formulations may help to limit metabolic complications.

Pharmacologic Therapy

Pharmacologic treatment of patients with CIPO aims to promote gastrointestinal propulsive activity, which may, in turn, improve oral feeding by decreasing severe symptoms, and reduce bacterial overgrowth related to intestinal stasis.

A variety of prokinetic drugs, eg, erythromycin, metoclopramide, domperidone (still not available in the United States), anticholinesterase drugs (neostigmine), serotoninergic agents (cisapride being the most effective one, but off the market since 1999 because of cardiac side effects), prostaglandins, somatostatin analogs (octreotide and lanreotide), and gonadotropin releasing hormone analogues (leuprolide) have been used with variable results in isolated cases or small series.[5,6,10] So far, only a few, mainly uncontrolled, trials have been published and the principal effects are summarized in **Table 3**.[60–66] A special mention should be made for the only 2 controlled studies which, however, date back to the 1990s. Notably, cisapride showed positive effects in accelerating gastric emptying and improving symptoms over placebo.[60,63] Among new serotoninergic drugs, prucalopride a highly selective serotonin $(5\text{-HT})_4$ receptor agonist with prominent enterokinetic effects[67] might be useful in patients with CIPO, although data for this drug in this indication are not, as yet, available. Empirical combinations of prokinetic drugs may be tried to increase their therapeutic effects and limit tachyphylaxis and side effects.

Cases of CIPO with histologically proved inflammatory neuropathy (ie, myenteric ganglionitis) may respond to immunosuppressive treatments.[29,36,39] Although promising, these results should be interpreted with extreme caution as only a few case reports have been published and data from controlled trials are still awaited.

Antibiotics should be used to treat bacterial overgrowth, an important cause of diarrhea and malnutrition in CIPO. Since breath tests and duodenal aspirate analysis are not sufficiently reliable, empirical trials with unabsorbable antibiotics, such as rifaximin, should be the treatment of choice.[68] Other antibiotics, however, such as metronidazole, ciprofloxacin, and doxycycline, may also be given in a rotating schedule.[51]

The treatment of secondary forms is aimed at the underlying pathologic conditions.

Surgical Therapy

In general, surgery has a limited role in the management of CIPO, although a few, extremely well characterized cases may be eligible for a surgical bypass or resection of the dysfunctional gastrointestinal segment. Of 9 patients (out of 21) with CIPO who underwent gastrointestinal bypass, 6 could be maintained on oral feeding.[69] A 20-year retrospective analysis of 8 cases of end-stage CIPO awaiting intestinal transplantation showed that a nearly total enterectomy proved to be an effective procedure in 6 patients, with 2 reporting a significant improvement.[70] However, due to the progressive nature in most cases of CIPO of the underlying gut dysfunction, the efficacy of surgery may be limited over time and prolonged postsurgical follow up studies have not been published. Gastrostomies and enterostomies are the most common surgical procedures in CIPO and can effectively relieve retching, vomiting, and abdominal distention.[71]

Transplantation

For patients with chronic intestinal failure and a high risk of mortality, life-threatening complications of TPN (including liver insufficiency and recurrent, intractable septicemia), lack of venous access for TPN, disease-related poor quality of life, despite optimal TPN, isolated or multivisceral intestinal transplantation have become an important therapeutic alternative.[59] Compared to cyclosporine, the use of new immunosuppressive agents, ie, tacrolimus, associated with steroids, and together with induction agents such as alemtuzumab, antilymphocyte globulins, and daclizumab, improved overall survival rates and decreased graft rejection rates.[72] According to one of the largest single-center published series of 98 consecutive patients who received multivisceral transplantation at the University of Miami, patient and graft survival rates, for all cases, were 49% and 47%, respectively, at 5 years.[73] Three factors were associated with poor prognosis: having undergone a transplant before 1998 (ie, prior to their introduction of multivisceral transplantation), being unable to stay out of the hospital before transplantation, and being a child.[73] Complications of small bowel transplantation include rejection, sepsis, a continued, long-term need for TPN and repeated laparotomies. Compared to other forms of intestinal failure, small bowel transplantation may be particularly challenging in CIPO patients because of a variety of factors including, concomitant neuromuscular disorders of the urinary tract, chronic use of opioids, and technical problems related to previous multiple laparotomies, and/or the need for gastrectomy for gastroparesis.

SUMMARY

CIPO is the very “tip of the iceberg” of functional gastrointestinal disorders, being a rare and frequently misdiagnosed condition characterized by an overall poor outcome. Diagnosis should be based on clinical features, natural history and radiologic findings. There is no cure for CIPO and management strategies include a wide array of nutritional, pharmacologic, and surgical options which are directed to minimize malnutrition, promote gut motility and reduce complications of stasis (ie, bacterial overgrowth). Pain may become so severe to necessitate major analgesic drugs.

Underlying causes of secondary CIPO should be thoroughly investigated and, if detected, treated accordingly. Surgery should be indicated only in a highly selected, well characterized subset of patients, while isolated intestinal or multivisceral transplantation is a rescue therapy only in those patients with intestinal failure unsuitable for or unable to continue with TPN/HPN. Future perspectives in CIPO will be directed toward an accurate genomic/proteomic phenotying of these rare, challenging patients. Unveiling causative mechanisms of neuro-ICC-muscular abnormalities will pave the way for targeted therapeutic options for patients with CIPO.

REFERENCES

1. Dudley HAF, Sinclair ISR, McLaren IF, et al. Intestinal pseudo-obstruction. J R Coll Surg Edin 1958;3:206–17.
2. Naish, JM, Capper WM, Brown NJ. Intestinal pseudo-obstruction with steatorrhoea. Gut 1960;1:62–6.
3. Stephens FO. The syndrome of intestinal pseudo-obstruction. Br J Med 1962;1: 1248–50.
4. Legge DA, Wollaeger EE, Carlson HC. Intestinal pseudo-obstruction in systemic amyloidosis. Gut 1970;11:764–7.
5. Stanghellini V, Corinaldesi R, Barbara L. Pseudo-obstruction syndromes. Baillieres Clin Gastroenterol 1988;2:225–54.
6. Di Lorenzo C. Pseudo-obstruction: current approaches. Gastroenterology 1999;116: 980–7.
7. De Giorgio R, Knowles CH. Acute colonic pseudo-obstruction. Br J Surg 2009;96: 229–39.
8. Stanghellini V, Camilleri M, Malagelada JR. Chronic idiopathic intestinal pseudo-obstruction: clinical and intestinal manometric findings. Gut 1987;28:5–12.
9. Stanghellini V, Cogliandro RF, De Giorgio R, et al. Natural history of chronic idiopathic intestinal pseudo-obstruction in adults: a single center study. Clin Gastroent Hepatol 2005;3:449–58.
10. Stanghellini V, Cogliandro RF, De Giorgio R, et al. Chronic intestinal pseudo-obstruction: manifestations, natural history and management. Neurogastroenterol Motil 2007;19:440–52.
11. Amiot A, Joly F, Alves A, et al. Long-term outcome of chronic intestinal pseudo-obstruction adult patients requiring home parenteral nutrition. Am J Gastroenterol 2009;104:1262–70.
12. Lindberg G, Iwarzon M, Tornblom H. Clinical features and long-term survival in chronic intestinal pseudo-obstruction and enteric dysmotility. Scand J Gastroenterol 2009; 44:692–9.
13. De Giorgio R, Stanghellini V, Barbara G, et al. Primary enteric neuropathies underlying gastrointestinal motor dysfunctions. Scand J Gastroenterol 2000;35:114–22.
14. De Giorgio R, Sarnelli G, Corinaldesi R, et al. Advance in our understanding of the pathology of chronic intestinal pseudo-obstruction. Gut 2004;53:1549–52.
15. De Giorgio R, Ricciardiello L, Naponelli V, et al. Chronic intestinal pseudo-obstruction related to viral infections. Transplant Proc 2010;42:9–14.
16. Stanghellini V, Corinaldesi R, Ghidini C, et al. Reversibility of gastrointestinal motor abnormalities in chronic intestinal pseudo-obstruction. Hepatogastroenterology 1992;39:34–8.
17. De Giorgio R, Seri M, Cogliandro R, et al. Analysis of candidate genes for intrinsic neuropathy in a family with chronic idiopathic intestinal pseudo-obstruction. Clin Gen 2001;59:131–3.

18. Pingault V, Guiochon-Mantel A, Bondurand N, et al. Peripheral neuropathy with hypomyelination, chronic intestinal pseudo-obstruction and deafness: a developmental "neural crest syndrome" related to a SOX10 mutation. Ann Neurol 2000;48:671–6.
19. Pingault V, Girard M, Bondurand N, et al. SOX10 mutations in chronic intestinal pseudo-obstruction suggest a complex physiopathological mechanism. Hum Genet 2002;111:198–206.
20. Mungan Z, Akyüz F, Bugra Z, et al. Familial visceral myopathy with pseudo-obstruction, megaduodenum, Barrett's esophagus, and cardiac abnormalities. Am J Gastroenterol 2003;98:2556–60.
21. Deglincerti A, De Giorgio R, Cefle K, et al. A novel locus for syndromic chronic idiopathic intestinal pseudo-obstruction maps to chromosome 8q23-q24. Eur J Hum Genet 2007;15:889–97.
22. Bardosi A, Creutzfeldt W, DiMauro S, et al. Myo-, neuro-, gastrointestinal encephalopathy (MNGIE syndrome) due to partial deficiency of cytochrome-c-oxidase. A new mitochondrial multisystem disorder. Acta Neuropathol 1987;74:248–58.
23. Nishino I, Spinazzola A, Hirano M. Thymidine phosphorylase gene mutations in MNGIE, a human mitochondrial disorder. Science 1999;283(5402):689–92.
24. Van Goethem G, Schwartz M, Lofgren A, et al. Novel POLG mutations in progressive external ophthalmoplegia mimicking mitochondrial neurogastrointestinal encephalomyopathy. Eur J Hum Genet 2003;11:547–9.
25. Giordano C, Sebastiani M, De Giorgio R, et al. Gastrointestinal dysmotility in mitochondrial neurogastrointestinal encephalomyopathy is caused by mitochondrial DNA depletion. Am J Pathol 2008;173:1120–8.
26. Gargiulo A, Auricchio R, Barone MV, et al. Filamin A is mutated in X-linked chronic idiopathic intestinal pseudo-obstruction with central nervous system involvement. Am J Hum Genet 2007;80:751–8.
27. Clayton-Smith J, Walters S, Hobson E, et al. Xq28 duplication presenting with intestinal and bladder dysfunction and a distinctive facial appearance. Eur J Hum Genet 2009;17:434–43.
28. Kapur RP, Robertson SP, Hannibal MC, et al. Diffuse abnormal layering of small intestinal smooth muscle is present in patients with FLNA mutations and X-linked intestinal pseudo-obstruction. Am J Surg Pathol 2010;34:1528–43.
29. De Giorgio R, Camilleri M. Human enteric neuropathies: morphology and molecular pathology. Neurogastroenterol Motil 2004;16:515–31.
30. Knowles CH, De Giorgio R, Kapur RP, et al. The London Classification of gastrointestinal neuromuscular pathology: report on behalf of the Gastro 2009 International Working Group. Gut 2010;59:882–7.
31. De Giorgio, Guerrini S, Barbara G, et al. Inflammatory neuropathies of the enteric nervous system. Gastroenterology 2004;126:1872–83.
32. Knowles CH, Silk DB, Darzi A, et al. Deranged smooth muscle alpha-actin as a biomarker of intestinal pseudo-obstruction: a controlled multinational case series. Gut 2004;53:1583–9.
33. Lindberg G, Törnblom H, Iwarzon M, et al. Full-thickness biopsy findings in chronic intestinal pseudo-obstruction and enteric dysmotility. Gut 2009;58:1084–90.
34. Veress B, Nyberg B, Törnblom H, et al. Intestinal lymphocytic epithelioganglionitis: a unique combination of inflammation in bowel dysmotility: a histopathological and immunohistochemical analysis of 28 cases. Histopathology 2009;54:539–49.
35. Knowles CH, De Giorgio R, Kapur RP, et al. Gastrointestinal neuromuscular pathology: guidelines for histological techniques and reporting on behalf of the Gastro 2009 International Working Group. Acta Neuropathol 2009;118:271–301.

36. De Giorgio R, Barbara G, Stanghellini V, et al. Clinical and morphofunctional features of idiopathic myenteric ganglionitis underlying severe intestinal motor dysfunction: a study of three cases. Am J Gastroenterol 2002;97:2454–9.
37. De Giorgio R, Bovara M, Barbara G, et al. Anti-HuD-induced neuronal apoptosis underlying paraneoplastic gut dysmotility. Gastroenterology 2003;125:70–9.
38. Hubball A, Martin JE, Lang B, et al. The role of humoral autoimmunity in gastrointestinal neuromuscular diseases. Prog Neurobiol 2009;87:10–20.
39. Di Nardo G, Blandizzi C, Volta U, et al. Review article: molecular, pathological and therapeutic features of human enteric neuropathies. Aliment Pharmacol Ther 2008;28:25–42.
40. Schäppi MG, Smith VV, Milla PJ, et al. Eosinophilic myenteric ganglionitis is associated with functional intestinal obstruction. Gut 2003;52:752–5.
41. Accarino A, Colucci R, Barbara G, et al. Mast cell neuromuscular involvement in patients with severe gastrointestinal dysmotility (SGID). Gut 2007;56(Suppl III):A18.
42. Mann SD, Debinski HS, Kamm MA. Clinical characteristics of chronic idiopathic intestinal pseudo-obstruction in adults. Gut 1997;41:675–81.
43. Bassotti G, Villanacci V. Can "functional" constipation be considered as a form of enteric neuro-gliopathy? Glia 201;59:345–50.
44. Oton E, Moreira V, Redondo C, et al. Chronic intestinal pseudoobstruction due to lymphocytic leiomyositis: is there a place for immunomodulatory therapy? Gut 2005;54:1343–4.
45. Dewit S, de Hertogh G, Geboes K, et al. Chronic intestinal pseudo-obstruction caused by an intestinal inflammatory myopathy: case report and review of the literature. Neurogastroenterol Motil 2008;20:343–8.
46. Smith JA, Hauser SC, Madara JL. Hollow visceral myopathy: a light- and electronmicroscopic study. Am J Surg Pathol 1982;6:269–75.
47. Schuffler MD. Chronic intestinal pseudo-obstruction syndromes. Med Clin North Am 1981;65:1331–58.
48. Wedel T, Van Eys GJ, Waltregny D, et al. Novel smooth muscle markers reveal abnormalities of the intestinal musculature in severe colorectal motility disorders. Neurogastroenterol Motil 2006;18:526–38.
49. Farrugia G. Interstitial cells of Cajal in health and disease. Neurogastroenterol Motil 2008;20 (Suppl 1):54–63.
50. Cogliandro RF, Antonucci A, De Giorgio R, et al. Patient-reported outcomes and gut dysmotility in functional gastrointestinal disorders. Neurogastroenterol Motil 2011, in press.
51. Lyford G, Foxx-Orenstein A. Chronic intestinal pseudo-obstruction. Curr Treat Options Gastroenterol 2004;7:317–25.
52. Lara MC, Valentino ML, Torres-Torronteras J, et al. Mitochondrial neurogastrointestinal encephalomyopathy (MNGIE): biochemical features and therapeutic approaches. Biosci Rep 2007;27:151–63.
53. Merlin A, Soyer P, Boudiaf M, et al. Chronic intestinal pseudo-obstruction in adult patients: multidetector row helical CT features. Eur Radiol 2008;18:1587–95.
54. Sumiyama K, Gostout CJ. Clinical applications of submucosal endoscopy. Curr Opin Gastroenterol 2011;27:412–7.
55. Kellow JE. Small intestine: normal function and clinical disorders. Manometry. In: Schuster MM, Crowell MD, Koch KL, editors. Schuster atlas of gastrointestinal motility in health and disease. Hamilton-London: BC Decker; 2002. p. 219–36.
56. Knowles CH, Veress B, Kapur RP, et al. Quantitation of cellular components of the enteric nervous system in the normal human gastrointestinal tract-report on behalf of the Gastro 2009 International Working Group. Neurogastroenterol Motil 2011;23:115–24.

57. Knowles CH, Veress B, Tornblom H, et al. Safety and diagnostic yield of laparoscopically assisted full-thickness bowel biospy. Neurogastroenterol Motil 2008;20:774–9.
58. Derkinderen P, Rouaud T, Lebouvier T, et al. Parkinson's disease: the enteric nervous system spills its guts. Neurology 2011, in press.
59. Pironi L, Spinucci G, Paganelli F, et al. Italian guidelines for intestinal transplantation: potential candidates among the adult patients managed by a medical referral center for chronic intestinal failure. Transplant Proc 2004;36:659–61.
60. Camilleri M, Malagelada JR, Abell TL, et al. Effect of six weeks of treatment with cisapride in gastroparesis and intestinal pseudo-obstruction. Gastroenterology 1989; 96:704–12.
61. Abell TL, Camilleri M, DiMagno EP, et al. Long-term efficacy of oral cisapride in symptomatic upper gut dysmotility. Dig Dis Sci 1991;36:616–20.
62. Soudah HC, Hasler WL, Owyang C. Effect of octreotide on intestinal motility and bacterial overgrowth in scleroderma. N Engl J Med 1991;325:1461–7.
63. Camilleri M, Balm RK, Zinsmeister AR. Determinant of response to a prokinetic agent in neuropathic chronic intestinal motility disorders. Gastroenterology 1994; 106:916–23.
64. Verne GN, Eaker EY, Hardy E, et al. Effect of octreotide and erythromycin on idiopathic and scleroderma-associated intestinal pseudoobstruction. Dig Dis Sci 1995;40:1892–901.
65. Camilleri M, Balm RK, Zinsmeister AR. Symptomatic improvement with one-year cisapride treatment in neuropathic chronic dysmotility. Aliment Pharmacol Ther 1996;10:403–9.
66. Emmanuel AV, Shand AG, Kamm MA. Erythromycin for the treatment of chronic intestinal pseudo-obstruction: description of six cases with a positive response. Aliment Pharmacol Ther 2004;19:687–94.
67. Sanger GJ. Translating 5-HT receptor pharmacology. Neurogastroenterol Motil 2009; 21:1235–8.
68. Pimentel M. Review of rifaximin as treatment for SIBO and IBS. Expert Opin Investig Drugs 2009;18:349–58.
69. Murr MM, Sarr MG, Camilleri M. The surgeon's role in the treatment of chronic intestinal pseudo-obstruction. Am J Gastroent 1995;90:2147–51.
70. Lapointe R. Chronic idiopathic intestinal pseudo-obstruction treated by near total small bowel resection: a 20-year experience. J Gastrointest Surg. 2010 Dec;14(12): 193742.
71. Pitt HA, Gomes AS, Lois JF, et al. Does preoperative percutaneous biliary drainage reduce operative risk or increase hospital cost? Ann Surg 1985;201:545–53.
72. Masetti M, Di Benedetto F, Cautero N, et al. Intestinal transplantation for chronic intestinal pseudo-obstruction in adult patients. Am J Transplantation 2004;4:826–9.
73. Tzakis AG, Kato T, Levi DM, et al. 100 multivisceral transplants at a single center. Ann Surg 2005;242:480–93.

Postoperative Problems 2011: Fundoplication and Obesity Surgery

W.O. Rohof, MD[a], R. Bisschops, MD, PhD[b], J. Tack, MD, PhD[c], G.E. Boeckxstaens, MD, PhD[c,*]

KEYWORDS

- Fundoplication • Bariatric surgery • Dysphagia
- Dumping syndrome • GERD

The population of the Western world is abundantly exposed to food. Together with the introduction of fast food, this situation has contributed to an exponential increase in morbid obesity.[1,2] Similarly, the prevalence of gastroesophageal reflux disease (GERD) has increased significantly in the past decades, representing one of the most common gastrointestinal (GI) disorders in the Western world.[3] The fact that morbid obesity is a significant risk factor for GERD certainly contributes to this tendency.

Neurogastroenterologists are mainly confronted with GERD patients presenting at the outpatient clinic or in the endoscopy room, often referred by the primary care physician with symptoms resistant to proton pump inhibitors (PPIs). With the introduction of laparoscopic surgery, however, more patients, especially younger patients or patients unwilling to take lifelong PPIs, are treated surgically. Although laparoscopic antireflux surgery is very effective in controlling reflux, the neurogastroenterologist is increasingly confronted with postsurgery complications; a similar situation now exists for obese patients who have undergone bariatric surgery. Weight reduction and GERD are, for the most part, effectively treated by the relevant surgical techniques used, but patients with symptoms resulting from abnormal motility secondary to altered anatomy or stenosis as a consequence of these procedures are increasingly presenting at our motility unit. In the current review, we will focus on the

The authors have nothing to disclose.

[a] Department of Gastroenterology and Hepatology, Academic Medical Center, Amsterdam, the Netherlands
[b] Department of Gastroenterology, University Hospital of Leuven and Catholic University of Leuven, Leuven, Belgium
[c] Department of Gastroenterology, Translational Research Center for Gastrointestinal Disorders (TARGID), University Hospital of Leuven and Catholic University of Leuven, Herestraat 49, 3000 Leuven, Belgium
* Corresponding author.
E-mail address: Guy.Boeckxstaens@med.kuleuven.be

Gastroenterol Clin N Am 40 (2011) 809–821
doi:10.1016/j.gtc.2011.09.002
0889-8553/11/$ – see front matter

postoperative complications of obesity surgery and fundoplication most commonly observed in the outpatient clinic.

OBESITY SURGERY

Obesity is a major medical problem that has seen such a dramatic increase in prevalence in the United States that it now exceeds 30% in both genders and in most age groups.[1,2] As obesity is a major risk factor for several serious medical conditions, such as arterial hypertension, cancer, diabetes, and cardiovascular diseases, this disorder should be rigorously treated.[4,5] Although different treatment modalities have been introduced, the best long-term results are currently obtained with obesity surgery.[4–6] For the most part, 1 of 3 different techniques is used to reduce food intake: laparoscopic adjustable gastric banding (LAGB), Roux-en-Y gastric bypass (RYGBP), and sleeve gastrectomy.

LAGB, introduced in 1993, is one of the most frequently performed surgical procedures to treat obesity worldwide, as it is a relatively simple to perform, minimal invasive and reversible. An inflatable device is positioned around the proximal stomach and then connected to a port reservoir, which is implanted 4 to 6 cm cranial to the xiphoid process and fixed to the periosteum of the sternum.[7,8] Approximately 4 weeks after surgery the band is filled with 2 to 4 ml of saline, thereby creating a small reservoir above the band, ensuring early satiation and reduced food intake. The volume is adjusted during follow-up so that, while solid food intolerance is avoided, food intake is reduced to approximately one-third to one-half of the volume ingested prior to surgery.[9] In the Roux-en-Y gastric bypass, the stomach is largely bypassed with only a small proximal gastric pouch remaining, while the stomach is drastically reduced in size by a sleeve gastrectomy.

In the early postsurgical period, complications such as leakage, infection, and bleeding can occur with all 3 procedures, but these are managed by the surgical team. Here, we will focus more on the long-term impact of these procedures on GI motility/physiology and the associated symptoms/complications, which will largely depend on the type of surgery to which the patient was exposed. Esophageal dysmotility disorders (dysphagia, esophageal dilatation, and heartburn [esophagitis])[10] are the main complications following LAGB, whereas dumping is the major complication of the 2 other techniques. These are the problems that the gastroenterologist is most likely to encounter.

Esophageal Dysmotility Disorders

In patients referred with dysphagia or heartburn following LAGB, displacement of the gastric band or an overinflated band should be excluded by imaging or endoscopy. A recent detailed analysis of a large series of patients (N = 167) treated with LAGB reported, indeed, that band deflation had to be carried out in approximately 30% (47 patients).[10] These patients presented with symptoms of solid food intolerance, nightly aspiration, and vomiting more than twice per week. On imaging, 7 patients had a hypercontractile esophagus, 34 had significant dilatation with anterior/posterior pouch slipping, and, most importantly, 6 patients presented with a major achalasia-like dilatation. The latter patients had to be reoperated on for band removal. Thus, radiographic evaluation of the position of the band and an estimation of transit through the esophagus are crucial. Data on esophageal motility assessed by esophageal manometry or impedance recordings, in this situation, are not available yet and are eagerly awaited.

The radiographic features described (ie, esophageal dilatation, hypercontractility [nutcracker-like esophagus], and, in the most advanced stage, an achalasia-like picture) most likely result from the chronically increased resistance that has to be overcome by the esophagus and are very similar to the situation created by a too-tight fundoplication (see later). Initially, the esophagus will try to overcome the resistance, resulting in a hypercontractile state, which will gradually "exhaust" the esophagus with resultant dilatation and, ultimately, an achalasia-like picture. Interestingly, following deflation or removal of the gastric band, esophageal dilatation has completely reversed.[10]

After gastric bypass, dysphagia can develop due to a stricture at the stoma in up to 19% of patients. Usually, it is advised to perform balloon dilation only up to 15 mm in diameter, in order to preserve the restrictive function of the RYGBP. In most patients, resolution of symptoms can be obtained with endoscopic treatment.[11]

Dumping Syndrome

The dumping syndrome is a well-described complication of both gastric bypass and sleeve gastrectomy and has also been documented, albeit less frequently, following esophageal surgery. This condition results from too rapid passage of food from the stomach into the small bowel.[12] Under normal conditions gastric emptying is tightly controlled through intimate coordination of motility of the proximal stomach, acting as a reservoir, and the distal stomach, where mixing and grinding result in the reduction of the ingested food into particles small enough to leave the stomach. The accommodation-reflex of the proximal stomach is a vagovagally mediated motor pattern that inhibits the tone of the proximal stomach, thereby creating a reservoir to temporarily store food.[13] Impaired relaxation of the proximal stomach results in early satiation and has been identified as an important pathophysiological mechanism in functional dyspepsia.[14] The main task of the distal stomach, on the other hand, is to gradually brake down food particles to a diameter of 1 to 2 mm, the critical size for passage through the pylorus and thus exiting the stomach. Finally, the pylorus, by acting as a gatekeeper controlling the outflow of the stomach, also significantly contributes to gastric emptying.

After upper GI surgery, such as a sleeve or partial gastrectomy, vagotomy, or even esophageal surgery, the absence of the vagovagal accommodation reflex and/or anatomical reduction of the size of the proximal stomach leads to an impaired reservoir function of the stomach and accelerated gastric emptying.[15–17] In the case of either a Roux-en-Y gastric bypass surgery or a resection of the distal stomach (Billroth I and II), the grinding activity of the antrum and the sifting function of the pylorus are eliminated resulting in the rapid arrival of large food particles in the small intestine. The increased exposure of the duodenum to these large, less easily digested, particles is considered to be the main pathophysiologic mechanism responsible for the development of the dumping syndrome after esophageal and, more frequently, gastric surgery.[12]

Typically, dumping symptoms can be divided into early (within 30 minutes) and late (1 to 3 hours after meal ingestion). Early symptoms are divided into GI complaints, such as abdominal pain, diarrhea, borborygmi, bloating, and nausea and the more specific vasomotor complaints such as flushing, palpitation, perspiration, tachycardia, hypotension, and even syncope. Early symptoms are probably a result of a fluid shift to the hyperosmolar duodenal lumen, resulting in a decrease of circulating volume and, thereby, to postprandial tachycardia, hypotension and, eventually, although rarely, syncope.[12,18] Additionally, the carbohydrate overload leads to a rapid release of GI peptide hormones that alter GI motility and can, in itself, also lead to the observed hemodynamic effects.[18–20] Late symptoms occur up to 3 hours postprandially and include hypoglycemia, perspiration, hunger, fatigue, and syncope. The excessive presentation of carbohydrates to the jejunum is thought to generate a rapid increase in insulin release via glucagon-like peptide (GLP-1), which eventually leads to hypoglycemia and related symptoms.[18,21]

The diagnosis of dumping syndrome is mainly based on clinical assessment and a modified oral glucose tolerance test. From 50 to 75 g of glucose solution is ingested after an overnight fast. Immediately before and up to 180 minutes after ingestion, blood glucose concentration, hematocrit, pulse rate, and blood pressure are recorded every 30 minutes. This provocative test is considered positive if late hypoglycemia (120 to 180 minutes) occurs or an early (30 minutes) rise in hematocrit (>3%) occurs. The best predictor of dumping, however, seems to be an increase in pulse rate (>10 bpm) after 30 minutes.[22] Assessment of accelerated gastric emptying can be helpful, but this test does not have good sensitivity and specificity.[18,22,23]

With the increased use of bariatric surgery, the incidence of dumping syndrome is rising; implying that clinicians should be familiar with the presentation and management of this syndrome. The first steps in the treatment of dumping syndrome are dietary measures. Patients are advised to eat more and smaller portions more frequently and to avoid drinking during the meal. Furthermore, the intake of fast-uptake carbohydrates should be limited. Most patients respond well to dietary measures, but for those who do not, acarbose is the next treatment step. Acarbose is an alpha-glycosidase hydrolase inhibitor that hinders the uptake of carbohydrates in the jejunum.[12,24] Small studies have indeed shown a reduction in hypoglycemia and an improvement in symptoms[24–27] (**Table 1**). However, because of its mechanism of action, acarbose is only helpful in patients with late dumping symptoms, as gastric emptying is unaffected. Furthermore, the frequent occurrence of side effects, such as bloating, flatulence, and diarrhea, hinder patient compliance. If patients fail to respond to acarbose, the next step is subcutaneous injection of somatostatin analogs, of which short-acting (octreotide) and long-acting (lanreotide, LAR) variants exist. Somatostatin analogs delay gastric emptying and small bowel transit and inhibit the release of GI hormones and insulin, and thus act on several pathophysiologic mechanisms involved in both the early and late phases of dumping. As a consequence, these agents have proven successful in the treatment of the postoperative dumping syndrome[23,28–34] (**Table 2**). As the long-acting variant has a confirmed effect on quality of life and is preferred by patients, monthly administration with LAR is indicated in patients with proven dietary-refractory dumping syndrome and impaired quality of life.[23,35] Known side effects, such as gallstone formation and steatorrhea, have to be considered in the decision on treatment.[23] If patients do not tolerate or do not respond to somatostatin analogues, surgery or continuous enteral feeding might be necessary but the results of these treatments are unpredictable.[12]

ANTIREFLUX SURGERY

Laparoscopic fundoplication is the recommended surgical therapy for GERD and is mainly used in patients who are unwilling to continue lifelong acid suppressive medication or who have experienced only partial therapeutic success. The first described, and most commonly used, is the Nissen fundoplication, in which a circumferential posterior wrap is made.[36] The Toupet fundoplication, on the other hand, creates a partial posterior wrap surrounding 270° of the esophagus.[37] Fundoplication has a high clinical success rate, even in patients with refractory symptoms to acid-suppressive medication, and in long-term follow-up.[38,39] In contrast to PPIs, both acid and weakly acid reflux episodes are reduced by fundoplication, most likely contributing to the excellent results reported.[40,41] However, postoperative symptoms

Table 1
Dumping syndrome studies

Study (year of publication)	No. of Patients	Treatment	Results
McLoughlin (1979)[24]	10	Acarbose 100 mg single administration before oral glucose tolerance test (OGTT)	Improvement of symptoms and attenuation of hypoglycemia during OGTT. Elevated plasma levels of gastric inhibitory polypeptide and insulin were reduced. No change in gastric emptying
Gerard (1983)[25]	24	Acarbose 100 mg single administration before OGTT	Attenuation of hypoglycemia during OGTT. Elevated plasma levels of insulin were reduced. Inhibition of sucrose-induced glucagon suppression
Lyons (1985)[26]	13	Acarbose 50 mg single administration before breakfast, continuation of therapy in 9 subjects	Attenuation of hypoglycemia. Elevated plasma levels of gastric inhibitory polypeptide, insulin, and enteroglucagon were reduced. Marked improvement in symptoms in some patients.
Hasegawa (1998)[27]	6	Acarbose 50–100 mg three times daily for a month	Attenuation of late dumping symptoms and glucose fluctuations. (uncontrolled)

Table 2
Controlled studies evaluating octreotide in dumping syndrome

Study (year of publication)	No. of Patients	Treatment	Results
Hopman (1988)[28]	12	Octreotide 50 μg vs placebo before OGTT	Improved dumping symptoms; suppression of postprandial rise in pulse rate; reduced peak insulin and increased nadir glycemia; delayed GI transit time
Primrose (1989)[29]	10	Octreotide 50 μg vs 100 μg vs placebo before OGTT	Reduced symptoms of early and late dumping; Attenuation of hypoglycemia; reduced pulse and systolic blood pressure changes
Tulassay (1989)[30]	8	Octreotide 50 μg vs placebo before OGTT	Improved dumping symptoms; no increase in insulin or gastric inhibitory polypeptide levels; suppression of rise in pulse and hematocrit
Geer (1990)[31]	10	Octreotide 100 μg vs placebo before a dumping provocative meal	Prevention of dumping symptoms, delayed gastric emptying and transit time, prevention of late hypoglycemia and of the rise in plasma levels of glucose, glucagon, pancreatic polypeptide, neurotensin and insulin.
Richards (1990)[32]	6	Octreotide 100 μg vs placebo before a dumping provocative meal	Prevention of dumping symptoms, fast induction of the migrating motor complex phase III in the duodenum
Gray (1991)[33]	9	Octreotide 100 μg vs placebo before a dumping provocative meal	Improvement of dumping symptoms, suppression of rise in hematocrit and pulse rate, inhibition of postprandial hypoglycemia
Hasler (1996)[34]	8	Octreotide 50 μg vs placebo before OGTT	Improvement of early and late dumping symptoms, suppression of rise in hematocrit and pulse rate, inhibition of postprandial hypoglycemia, no influence on gastric emptying rate
Arts (2009)[23]	30	Octreotide 50 μg vs placebo before OGTT	Improvement of early and late dumping symptoms, suppression of rise in hematocrit and pulse rate, inhibition of postprandial hypoglycemia.

such as dysphagia, bloating, flatulence, and the inability to belch are common and probably underreported.

Dysphagia

In a recent meta-analysis, the 2 most commonly used surgical antireflux techniques, total and partial fundoplication, were compared. Interestingly, partial fundoplication was associated with a significant reduction in the rates for postoperative dysphagia, dilatations for dysphagia, and surgical reinterventions compared to a total fundoplication, whereas the degree of symptom control, as well as rates of esophagitis and esophageal acid exposure, were similar for both treatments.[38] Therefore, the authors concluded that a partial fundoplication is the surgical antireflux procedure of choice for patients with GERD and, particularly in patients with abnormal preoperative manometry.

After fundoplication, early postoperative dysphagia occurs in up to 15% to 20% of patients, likely due to functional esophagogastric junction (EGJ) obstruction as a result of manipulation, local edema or hematoma.[38,42–45] Conservative measures such as supplemental feeding, dietary measures and reassurance are usually advocated, since symptoms resolve in most. More important is dysphagia, mostly for solids, persisting for longer than 2 to 3 months after surgery. Studies report that up to 10% of patients have persistent dysphagia that requires additional therapy.

The presence of preoperative esophageal motor dysfunction has been proposed to be predictive of the occurrence of postoperative dysphagia. Therefore, tailoring the degree of fundoplication according to status of preoperative esophageal motility has been advocated for a long time.[46–48] However, multiple studies have failed to demonstrate that preoperative manometry findings are a predictor of postoperative dysphagia or of the likelihood of reintervention for dysphagia after fundoplication.[43,48,49]

If patients present with persisting dysphagia, diagnostic evaluation is indicated.[42,49,50] A barium swallow and endoscopic evaluation are used to estimate the degree of stasis/stenosis and evaluate the intactness and position of the wrap. Anatomical abnormalities that can cause postoperative dysphagia are a too-tight wrap, displacement of the wrap (slipped Nissen), or hiatal fibrosis or stenosis; frequently no abnormalities are found.[51] Rarely, patients with achalasia misdiagnosed as GERD have been treated by a fundoplication.[52] Postoperative manometry should therefore be performed in patients in whom a preoperative examination is lacking. High-resolution esophageal manometry, on the other hand, is useful to demonstrate an elevated intrabolus pressure, indicative of EGJ obstruction.[53,54]

Interventions with proven treatment success are dilation and reoperation, indicated in 7% and 3% of patients after fundoplication, respectively.[49,55] Patients with anatomic abnormalities such as a slipped wrap should be considered for surgery early, but otherwise, dilations should be attempted first.[50] Dilations can be performed with bougies or through-the-scope balloons. Bougies and through-the-scope Rigiflex balloons range up to 20 mm in maximal diameter and are a safe and effective treatment option, particularly in patients without anatomic or manometric abnormalities.[50,56–58] Initial pneumatic dilation is performed with the minimal balloon volume of 30 mm, and has a success rate of 56% to 64%, although only studies of small sample size are available[56,57,59–61] (**Table 3**). If these endoscopic procedures are unsuccessful, surgical revision is indicated and is required in 3% to 6% of patients to resolve dysphagia.[55,62] It has to be emphasized though, that morbidity, treatment failure rates, and surgical complications are higher for redo surgery compared to the initial procedure, due to adhesions and the altered surgical anatomy. Nevertheless,

Table 3
Success rate of pneumatic dilation in postfundoplication dysphagia

Study (year of publication)	No. of Patients	Dilation Technique and Degree of Inflation (mm)	Success Rate	Serious Adverse Events
Gaudric (2001)[59]	16	Rigiflex balloon to 35 to 40 mm	9 of 16 (56%)	
Fumagalli (2007)[61]	8	Not specified	5 of 8 (63%)	
Hui (2002)[56]	14	Rigiflex balloon to 30 to 35 to 40 mm	9 of 14 (64%)	
Ellingson (1995)[60]	8	Rigiflex balloon to 30 to 35 to 40	5 of 8 (63%)	One perforation occurred, requiring surgery
Total	46		28 of 46 (61%)	

reoperation is still quite successful with success rates of 70% to 80%, most likely as these procedures are preferably performed in tertiary referral centers.[50,51,55]

Gas-Bloat Syndrome

The combination of bloating, the inability to belch, and flatulence are typical in the gas-bloat syndrome, observed in up to 20% of patients after fundoplication.[41,63] These symptoms are caused by the consequent reduction in the frequency of transient lower esophageal sphincter relaxations (TLESRs). This motor pattern is characterized by a prolonged absence of lower esophageal sphincter tone, accompanied by an inhibition of the crural diaphragm, and is widely recognized to be the major underlying pathophysiologic mechanism of GERD. However, as TLESRs are also the physiologic mechanism whereby one normally vents gas from the stomach, there is an increased risk for gas accumulation in the stomach following antireflux surgery.[40,64] Studies with pH-impedance before and after surgery have indeed demonstrated that fundoplication reduces the rate of gastric belches by 65%.[65] However, the frequency of supragastric belches is increased to a similar extent. Therefore, most patients probably do not notice the inability to belch or even report increased belching.[65]

Treatment is generally not necessary, and the number of affected patients declines with prolonged follow-up. Nevertheless, no evidence-based treatment is currently available for these patients, except for surgical revision. Partial fundoplication does lead to fewer symptoms of bloating and complaints of an inability to belch compared to complete fundoplication.[38]

Recurrent Reflux Symptoms

Long-term success rates for antireflux surgery vary between 85% and 90%.[62,66] However, studies have reported a high need for acid suppressive medication after a long period of follow-up: up to 62% in one study.[67] Risk factors for recurrent reflux symptoms after fundoplication are a high level of supine esophageal acid exposure and poor esophageal peristalsis before treatment.[68]

When a patient presents with recurrent reflux symptoms, it is important to objectively determine the relation between reflux episodes and symptoms. The gold standard is the ambulatory pH-impedance recording, as it detects pathologic acid exposure and also provides an assessment of the correlation between symptoms and acid or nonacid reflux events.[69] If neither acid exposure nor a significant symptom association is detected, the diagnosis of functional heartburn is suspected, and empirical therapy with a low dose of tricyclic antidepressant as a pain modulator can be attempted.[69] When recurrent symptoms are due to reflux, acid-suppressive medication combined with baclofen should be considered. This compound has repeatedly been shown to reduce both acid and nonacid reflux, even in PPI-resistant patients.[70,71] Only in patients unresponsive to any of these measures should surgical reintervention be considered, but, as noted before, this will be more difficult than the initial procedure due to adhesions and the presence of an altered surgical anatomy.

Early Satiety and Dyspeptic Symptoms, Dumping Syndrome

As outlined earlier, the proximal stomach acts as a reservoir accommodating ingested food. During antireflux surgery, the fundus is wrapped around the esophagus to prevent reflux. The downside of this procedure, however, is that the reservoir function of the stomach is impaired. In addition, damage to the vagus nerve is a well known complication of antireflux surgery,[72] further contributing to impaired accommodation of the proximal stomach. Functional studies have confirmed the presence of impaired accommodation following antireflux surgery.[73] As this abnormality is associated with early satiety,[14] these findings most likely explain the development of dyspeptic symptoms, especially early satiety, following antireflux surgery. It should be emphasized that a considerable proportion of patients may already have complained of dyspeptic symptoms before surgery but, quite often, these symptoms have not been adequately elicited or assessed. Obviously, patient selection is of crucial importance to prevent the performance of surgery on patients with functional complaints. This is definitely a major clinical challenge, not only in daily practice but also for investigators studying clinical efficacy of new antireflux compounds.

Finally, although less seen frequently than after gastric surgery, dumping syndrome can develop following antireflux surgery, most likely due to the reduction in proximal stomach volume and injury to the vagus nerve.

SUMMARY

Although the surgical treatment of both GERD and obesity is very successful, these procedures have a significant impact on the physiology and function of the proximal GI tract. With the increasing prevalence of both GERD and obesity, more and more patients present at the motility outpatient clinic with symptoms related to surgical interventions for these medical problems. In this review, we describe the main complications following antireflux surgery: dysphagia, gas bloat syndrome, recurrent (persistent) GERD symptoms, and dyspeptic symptoms. The most common motility-related complications of obesity surgery are dumping syndrome and esophageal dysmotility.

REFERENCES

1. Ogden CL, Carroll MD, Curtin LR, et al. Prevalence of overweight and obesity in the United States, 1999–2004. JAMA 2006;295:1549–55.
2. Nguyen DM, El-Serag HB. The epidemiology of obesity. Gastroenterol Clin North Am 2010;39:1–7.
3. Dent J, El-Serag HB, Wallander MA, et al. Epidemiology of gastro-oesophageal reflux disease: a systematic review. Gut 2005;54:710–7.
4. Sjostrom L, Lindroos AK, Peltonen M, et al. Lifestyle, diabetes, and cardiovascular risk factors 10 years after bariatric surgery. N Engl J Med 2004;351:2683–93.

5. Sjostrom L, Gummesson A, Sjostrom CD, et al. Effects of bariatric surgery on cancer incidence in obese patients in Sweden (Swedish Obese Subjects Study): a prospective, controlled intervention trial. Lancet Oncol 2009;10:653–62.
6. Sjostrom L, Narbro K, Sjostrom CD, et al. Effects of bariatric surgery on mortality in Swedish obese subjects. N Engl J Med 2007;357:741–52.
7. Catona A, Gossenberg M, La MA, et al. Laparoscopic gastric banding: preliminary series. Obes Surg 1993;3:207–9.
8. Wright TA, Kow L, Wilson T, et al. Early results of laparoscopic Swedish adjustable gastric banding for morbid obesity. Br J Surg 2000;87:362–73.
9. Naef M, Naef U, Mouton WG, et al. Outcome and complications after laparoscopic Swedish adjustable gastric banding: 5-year results of a prospective clinical trial. Obes Surg 2007;17:195–201.
10. Naef M, Mouton WG, Naef U, et al. Esophageal dysmotility disorders after laparoscopic gastric banding: an underestimated complication. Ann Surg 2011; 253:285–90.
11. Huang CS, Forse RA, Jacobson BC, et al. Endoscopic findings and their clinical correlations in patients with symptoms after gastric bypass surgery. Gastrointest Endosc 2003;58:859–66.
12. Tack J, Arts J, Caenepeel P, et al. Pathophysiology, diagnosis and management of postoperative dumping syndrome. Nat Rev Gastroenterol Hepatol 2009;6:583–90.
13. Tack J. Gastric motor and sensory function. Curr Opin Gastroenterol 2009;25: 557–65.
14. Tack J, Piessevaux H, Coulie B, et al. Role of impaired gastric accommodation to a meal in functional dyspepsia. Gastroenterology 1998;115:1346–52.
15. Abell TL, Minocha A. Gastrointestinal complications of bariatric surgery: diagnosis and therapy. Am J Med Sci 2006;331:214–8.
16. Zaloga GP, Chernow B. Postprandial hypoglycemia after Nissen fundoplication for reflux esophagitis. Gastroenterology 1983;84:840–2.
17. Mayer EA, Thompson JB, Jehn D, et al. Gastric emptying and sieving of solid food and pancreatic and biliary secretion after solid meals in patients with truncal vagotomy and antrectomy. Gastroenterology 1982;83(1 Pt 2):184–92.
18. Vecht J, Masclee AA, Lamers CB. The dumping syndrome. Current insights into pathophysiology, diagnosis and treatment. Scand J Gastroenterol Suppl 1997;223: 21–7.
19. Bloom SR, Royston CM, Thomson JP. Enteroglucagon release in the dumping syndrome. Lancet 1972;2(7781):789–91.
20. Lawaetz O, Blackburn AM, Bloom SR, et al. Gut hormone profile and gastric emptying in the dumping syndrome. A hypothesis concerning the pathogenesis. Scand J Gastroenterol 1983;18:73–80.
21. Toft-Nielsen M, Madsbad S, Holst JJ. Exaggerated secretion of glucagon-like peptide-1 (GLP-1) could cause reactive hypoglycaemia. Diabetologia 1998;41:1180–6.
22. van der Kleij FG, Vecht J, Lamers CB, et al. Diagnostic value of dumping provocation in patients after gastric surgery. Scand J Gastroenterol 1996;31:1162–6.
23. Arts J, Caenepeel P, Bisschops R, et al. Efficacy of the long-acting repeatable formulation of the somatostatin analogue octreotide in postoperative dumping. Clin Gastroenterol Hepatol 2009;7:432–7.
24. McLoughlin JC, Buchanan KD, Alam MJ. A glycoside-hydrolase inhibitor in treatment of dumping syndrome. Lancet 1979;2(8143):603–5.
25. Gerard J, Luyckx AS, Lefebvre PJ. Acarbose in reactive hypoglycemia: a double-blind study. Int J Clin Pharmacol Ther Toxicol 1984;22:25–31.

26. Lyons TJ, McLoughlin JC, Shaw C, et al. Effect of acarbose on biochemical responses and clinical symptoms in dumping syndrome. Digestion 1985;31(2-3): 89–96.
27. Hasegawa T, Yoneda M, Nakamura K, et al. Long-term effect of alpha-glucosidase inhibitor on late dumping syndrome. J Gastroenterol Hepatol 1998;13:1201–6.
28. Hopman WP, Wolberink RG, Lamers CB, et al. Treatment of the dumping syndrome with the somatostatin analogue SMS 201-995. Ann Surg 1988;207:155–9.
29. Primrose JN, Johnston D. Somatostatin analogue SMS 201-995 (octreotide) as a possible solution to the dumping syndrome after gastrectomy or vagotomy. Br J Surg 1989;76:140–4.
30. Tulassay Z, Tulassay T, Gupta R, et al. Long acting somatostatin analogue in dumping syndrome. Br J Surg 1989;76:1294–5.
31. Geer RJ, Richards WO, O'Dorisio TM, et al. Efficacy of octreotide acetate in treatment of severe postgastrectomy dumping syndrome. Ann Surg 1990;212:678–87.
32. Richards WO, Geer R, O'Dorisio TM, et al. Octreotide acetate induces fasting small bowel motility in patients with dumping syndrome. J Surg Res 1990;49:483–7.
33. Gray JL, Debas HT, Mulvihill SJ. Control of dumping symptoms by somatostatin analogue in patients after gastric surgery. Arch Surg 1991;126:1231–5.
34. Hasler WL, Soudah HC, Owyang C. Mechanisms by which octreotide ameliorates symptoms in the dumping syndrome. J Pharmacol Exp Ther 1996;277:1359–65.
35. Didden P, Penning C, Masclee AA. Octreotide therapy in dumping syndrome: analysis of long-term results. Aliment Pharmacol Ther 2006;24:1367–75.
36. Nissen R. [A simple operation for control of reflux esophagitis]. Schweiz Med Wochenschr 1956;86(Suppl 20):590–2.
37. Toupet A. [Technic of esophago-gastroplasty with phrenogastropexy used in radical treatment of hiatal hernias as a supplement to Heller's operation in cardiospasms]. Mem Acad Chir (Paris) 1963;89:384–9.
38. Broeders JA, Mauritz FA, Ahmed AU, et al. Systematic review and meta-analysis of laparoscopic Nissen (posterior total) versus Toupet (posterior partial) fundoplication for gastro-oesophageal reflux disease. Br J Surg 2010;97:1318–30.
39. Mardani J, Lundell L, Engstrom C. Total or posterior partial fundoplication in the treatment of GERD: results of a randomized trial after 2 decades of follow-up. Ann Surg 2011;253:875–8.
40. Bredenoord AJ, Draaisma WA, Weusten BL, et al. Mechanisms of acid, weakly acidic and gas reflux after anti-reflux surgery. Gut 2008;57:161–6.
41. Broeders JA, Bredenoord AJ, Hazebroek EJ, et al. Effects of anti-reflux surgery on weakly acidic reflux and belching. Gut 2011;60:435–41.
42. Bais JE, Bartelsman JF, Bonjer HJ, et al. Laparoscopic or conventional Nissen fundoplication for gastro-oesophageal reflux disease: randomised clinical trial. The Netherlands Antireflux Surgery Study Group. Lancet 2000;355(9199):170–4.
43. Strate U, Emmermann A, Fibbe C, et al. Laparoscopic fundoplication: Nissen versus Toupet two-year outcome of a prospective randomized study of 200 patients regarding preoperative esophageal motility. Surg Endosc 2008;22:21–30.
44. Mickevicius A, Endzinas Z, Kiudelis M, et al. Influence of wrap length on the effectiveness of Nissen and Toupet fundoplication: a prospective randomized study. Surg Endosc 2008;22:2269–76.
45. Lundell L. Complications after anti-reflux surgery. Best Pract Res Clin Gastroenterol 2004;18:935–45.
46. Hunter JG, Swanstrom L, Waring JP. Dysphagia after laparoscopic antireflux surgery. The impact of operative technique. Ann Surg 1996;224:51–7.

47. Gill RC, Bowes KL, Murphy PD, et al. Esophageal motor abnormalities in gastro-esophageal reflux and the effects of fundoplication. Gastroenterology 1986;91:364–9.
48. Tsuboi K, Lee TH, Legner A, et al. Identification of risk factors for postoperative dysphagia after primary anti-reflux surgery. Surg Endosc 2011;25:923–9.
49. Broeders JA, Sportel IG, Jamieson GG, et al. Impact of ineffective oesophageal motility and wrap type on dysphagia after laparoscopic fundoplication. Br J Surg 2011.
50. Sayuk GS, Clouse RE. Management of esophageal symptoms following fundoplication. Curr Treat Options Gastroenterol 2005;8:293–303.
51. Furnee EJ, Draaisma WA, Broeders IA, et al. Surgical reintervention after antireflux surgery for gastroesophageal reflux disease: a prospective cohort study in 130 patients. Arch Surg 2008;143:267–74.
52. Kessing B, Bredenoord AJ, Smout AJ. Erroneous Diagnosis of Gastroesophageal Reflux Disease in Achalasia. Clin Gastroenterol Hepatol 2011.
53. Scheffer RC, Samsom M, Haverkamp A, et al. Impaired bolus transit across the esophagogastric junction in postfundoplication dysphagia. Am J Gastroenterol 2005;100:1677–84.
54. Pandolfino JE, Ghosh SK, Lodhia N, et al. Utilizing intraluminal pressure gradients to predict esophageal clearance: a validation study. Am J Gastroenterol 2008;103:1898–905.
55. Lamb PJ, Myers JC, Jamieson GG, et al. Long-term outcomes of revisional surgery following laparoscopic fundoplication. Br J Surg 2009;96:391–7.
56. Hui JM, Hunt DR, de Carle DJ, et al. Esophageal pneumatic dilation for postfundoplication dysphagia: safety, efficacy, and predictors of outcome. Am J Gastroenterol 2002;97:2986–91.
57. Wo JM, Trus TL, Richardson WS, et al. Evaluation and management of postfundoplication dysphagia. Am J Gastroenterol 1996;91:2318–22.
58. Malhi-Chowla N, Gorecki P, Bammer T, et al. Dilation after fundoplication: timing, frequency, indications, and outcome. Gastrointest Endosc 2002;55:219–23.
59. Gaudric M, Sabate JM, Artru P, et al. Results of pneumatic dilatation in patients with dysphagia after antireflux surgery. Br J Surg 1999;86:1088–91.
60. Ellingson TL, Kozarek RA, Gelfand MD, et al. Iatrogenic achalasia. A case series. J Clin Gastroenterol 1995;20:96–9.
61. Fumagalli U, Bona S, Battafarano F, et al. Persistent dysphagia after laparoscopic fundoplication for gastro-esophageal reflux disease. Dis Esophagus 2008;21:257–61.
62. Broeders JA, Rijnhart-de Jong HG, Draaisma WA, et al. Ten-year outcome of laparoscopic and conventional nissen fundoplication: randomized clinical trial. Ann Surg 2009;250:698–706.
63. Pessaux P, Arnaud JP, Delattre JF, et al. Laparoscopic antireflux surgery: five-year results and beyond in 1340 patients. Arch Surg 2005;140:946–51.
64. Lindeboom MA, Ringers J, Straathof JW, et al. Effect of laparoscopic partial fundoplication on reflux mechanisms. Am J Gastroenterol 2003;98:29–34.
65. Broeders JA, Bredenoord AJ, Hazebroek EJ, et al. Effects of anti-reflux surgery on weakly acidic reflux and belching. Gut 2011;60:435–41.
66. Galmiche JP, Hatlebakk J, Attwood S, et al. Laparoscopic antireflux surgery vs esomeprazole treatment for chronic GERD: the LOTUS randomized clinical trial. JAMA 2011;305:1969–77.

67. Spechler SJ. Comparison of medical and surgical therapy for complicated gastroesophageal reflux disease in veterans. The Department of Veterans Affairs Gastroesophageal Reflux Disease Study Group. N Engl J Med 1992;326:786–92.
68. Broeders JA, Roks DJ, Draaisma WA, et al. Predictors of objectively identified recurrent reflux after primary Nissen fundoplication. Br J Surg 2011;98:673–9.
69. Fass R, Sifrim D. Management of heartburn not responding to proton pump inhibitors. Gut 2009;58:295–309.
70. Vela MF, Tutuian R, Katz PO, et al. Baclofen decreases acid and non-acid postprandial gastro-oesophageal reflux measured by combined multichannel intraluminal impedance and pH. Aliment Pharmacol Ther 2003;17:243–51.
71. Koek GH, Sifrim D, Lerut T, et al. Effect of the GABA(B) agonist baclofen in patients with symptoms and duodeno-gastro-oesophageal reflux refractory to proton pump inhibitors. Gut 2003;52:1397–402.
72. Lindeboom MY, Ringers J, van Rijn PJ, et al. Gastric emptying and vagus nerve function after laparoscopic partial fundoplication. Ann Surg 2004;240:785–90.
73. Bredenoord AJ, Chial HJ, Camilleri M, et al. Gastric accommodation and emptying in evaluation of patients with upper gastrointestinal symptoms. Clin Gastroenterol Hepatol 2003;1:264–72.

Challenges in the Swallowing Mechanism: Nonobstructive Dysphagia in the Era of High-Resolution Manometry and Impedance

Sabine Roman, MD, PhD[a,b], Peter J. Kahrilas, MD, AGAF[a,*]

KEYWORDS

- Dysphagia • High-resolution manometry • Impedance
- Esophagogastric junction

Esophageal motility disorders may be an explanation of dysphagia in patients after exclusion of esophageal structural lesions by endoscopy and radiography and eosinophilic esophagitis by histology. The best defined motility disorder is achalasia; however, other motility disorders such as diffuse esophageal spasm (DES), hypercontractile esophagus, and absent or weak peristalsis have also been reported with dysphagia.[1]

Esophageal manometry characterizes the contractility of the esophagus to identify and classify motility disorders. High-resolution manometry (HRM) with esophageal pressure topography (EPT) analysis is now the method of choice to assess esophageal contractile function.[2] These techniques were initially described by Clouse in the 1990s.[3] The concept of HRM is to overcome the limitations of conventional manometric systems by using advanced electronic technologies. The key to this development involved vastly increasing the number of pressure sensors on the manometric assembly. Pressure sensors are placed with sufficient proximity to each other so that, by interpolating between adjacent sensors, intraluminal pressure can be viewed as a continuum along the length of the entire esophagus and adjacent sphincters. When HRM is coupled with improved sensor design, such that each sensor is circumferentially sensitive and capable of high-fidelity recordings, it also overcomes the fidelity

This work was supported by Grant No. R01DK56033 from the National Institutes of Health.
Sabine Roman has served as a consultant for Given Imaging.
[a] Northwestern University, Department of Medicine, Feinberg School of Medicine, 676 St. Clair Street, Chicago, IL 60611, USA
[b] Digestive Physiology Department, Claude Bernard Lyon I University and Hospices Civils de Lyon, Pavillon H, 5 place d'Arsonval, F-69437 Lyon Cedex 03, France
* Corresponding author.
E-mail address: p-kahrilas@northwestern.edu

Gastroenterol Clin N Am 40 (2011) 823–835
doi:10.1016/j.gtc.2011.09.006
gastro.theclinics.com

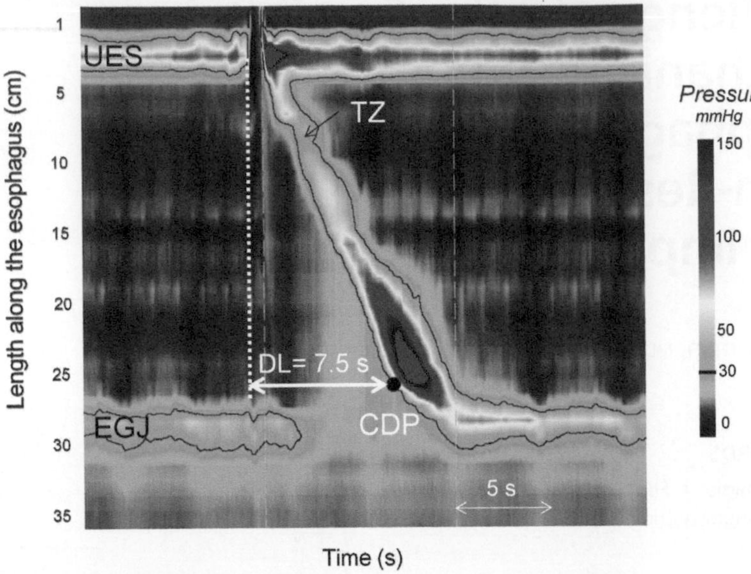

Fig. 1. EPT plot of normal swallow. The black line represents the 30 mm Hg IBC. Before swallowing, two high-pressure zones are visualized: the UES and the EGJ. During swallowing, the pharyngeal contraction wave occurs and UES pressure decreases. In the esophageal body, swallowing induces first a period of latency followed by peristaltic esophageal contraction. The proximal third of peristaltic esophageal contraction is separated from the distal two thirds by the transition zone (TZ). The CDP (*black dot*) represents the inflexion point in the contractile front propagation. The EGJ relaxation starts just after swallowing. DL is measured from the onset of UES relaxation to the CDP.

and directionality limitations inherent in conventional water-perfused systems. The final technological advance that facilitated the widespread application of HRM to clinical manometry was the development of sophisticated plotting algorithms to display the hugely expanded manometric data set as colored EPT plots rather than as a multitude of overlapping line tracings.[3,4] Together, these developments facilitate dynamic imaging of intraesophageal pressure as a continuum along the length of the esophagus with pressure magnitude depicted by spectral color. **Fig. 1** depicts the typical pressure topography of both sphincters and the entire length of intervening esophagus during a swallow. The relative timing of sphincter relaxation, segmental esophageal contraction, as well as the position and length of pressure troughs between segments, are all readily demonstrated.

The use of intraluminal impedance to monitor the bolus movement within the gastrointestinal (GI) tract was first described by Silny in 1991.[5] The technique is based on measurement of electrical impedance between closely placed electrodes mounted on an intraluminal probe. Impedance between each electrode pair depends on the nature of the luminal contents surrounding the electrodes. When the esophagus is empty, the impedance reflects the conductivity of the esophageal mucosa. Otherwise, it is indicative of surrounding intraluminal air (high impedance) or liquid (low impedance). With multiple pairs of impedance rings along the lumen of the esophagus, the spatial distribution and movement of air or liquid within the esophagus can be detected. Validation studies have verified that intraluminal impedance measurement has a high sensitivity and accuracy for tracking intraesophageal bolus movement and monitoring reflux.[6,7] However, it is important to note that the technique is not sensitive to the volume of the bolus or refluxate; 1.0 mL of residue potentially yields the same signal as 10 mL.[8]

In conjunction with HRM, impedance monitoring allows tracking the swallowed bolus in relation to EPT. Although the impedance data are ideally also displayed in a topographic format, the validated criteria for bolus presence within a segment is of a 50% decrease in impedance while a 50% increase toward the baseline value correlates with bolus exit.[9] Swallows can then be classified as having complete bolus transit if bolus entry is seen at the most proximal site and bolus exit is recorded in all distal impedance-measuring sites, or incomplete bolus transit, if bolus exit is not identified at one or more of the distal impedance-measuring sites.[10]

ACHALASIA

Achalasia is both the best-defined esophageal motor disorder and the one with the most specific treatment, making its accurate identification a key objective of clinical manometry. The manometric criteria for diagnosing achalasia are incomplete lower esophageal sphincter (LES) relaxation and absent peristalsis.[11] One of the greatest gains realized with HRM over conventional manometry has been in refining the definition of both of these criteria, with the net effect of greatly improved accuracy in the identification of the varied contractile patterns of achalasia.

It is a common misconception that the LES (esophagogastric junction [EGJ]) normally relaxes completely to intragastric pressure after swallowing. In fact, this is distinctly unusual and even abnormal. Rather, the EGJ relaxes to a value that is close to intragastric pressure for a certain amount of time during the post-deglutitive period. Considerable effort has been expended in using EPT to define more precisely these vague terms of "close to intragastric pressure" and "certain amount of time." Deglutitive EGJ relaxation occurs at a fixed time and place on EPT plots. **Fig. 2** illustrates the location and relaxation of the sphincter during bolus transit relative to the pharyngeal swallow. In most instances, EGJ relaxation is measured in the region spanning from 2 cm above the proximal aspect of the EGJ at rest to the proximal stomach for a 10-second period commencing with upper esophageal sphincter (UES) relaxation. In the setting of normal peristalsis, the window terminates with the arrival of the peristaltic contraction, but in the setting of failed peristalsis, an arbitrary 10-second cutoff is established, and in the setting of a premature distal esophageal contraction, a very brief window of opportunity exists. Note that if sphincter elevation exceeds 2 cm, as evident by the position of the LES during the post-deglutitive contraction, the spatial limits for the measurement need to be adjusted accordingly. Once the spatial limits of the EGJ relaxation window are established, maximal EGJ pressure is then ascertained for each instant within the window—in essence, an e-sleeve measurement. The resultant data set then amounts to a history of EGJ residual pressure commencing at the instant of UES relaxation and ending either with the arrival of the esophageal contraction or 10 seconds later. However, it is overly simplistic to think of EGJ relaxation pressure as solely indicative of LES relaxation. Actually, at any one instant the e-sleeve pressure is the greatest of three possible contributions: LES pressure, crural diaphragm contraction, or intrabolus pressure as the swallowed water traverses the EGJ. Hence, the development of the EPT relaxation metric of the integrated relaxation pressure (IRP).[12] The IRP is measured within the deglutitive window, capturing the axial movement of the LES and spanning from the time of initiation of the swallow until the arrival of the peristaltic contraction with the added stipulation that the relaxation pressure being reported represents the 4-second period of lowest EGJ pressure after the swallow (see **Fig. 2**). **Table 1**

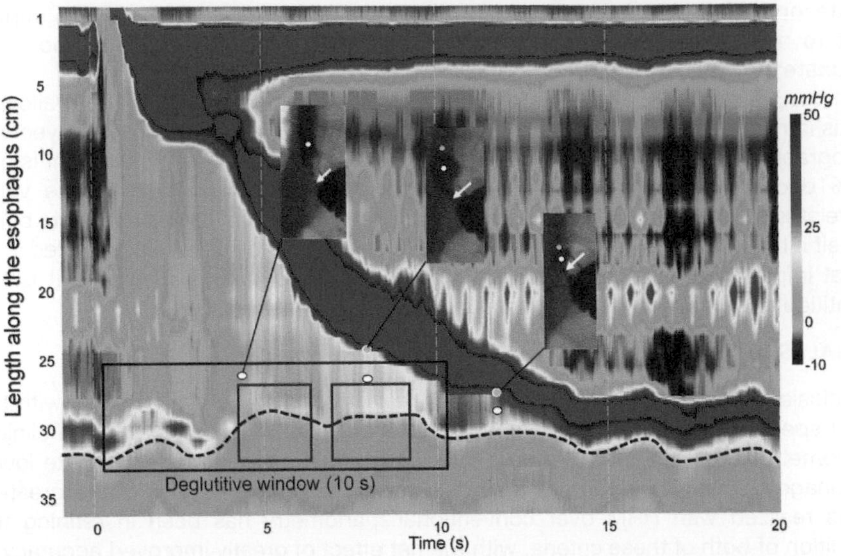

Fig. 2. Concomitant EPT and fluoroscopy during esophageal emptying. The fluoroscopic images in the windows are synchronized with the EPT plot. The white and blue dots indicate areas of intrabolus pressure and the onset of luminal closure, respectively. The second image (at about time 8 seconds) is near the CDP, evident both by the transition of the fluoroscopic image to ampullary conformation and slowing of the luminal closure front. The maroon rectangles within the deglutitive relaxation window (*black rectangle*) indicate the time fragments used to compute the IRP. The distal border of the EGJ is indicated by black dashed line on EPT and by white arrows on barium swallow.

illustrates the added yield of the IRP compared to the nadir LES or EGJ pressure in the detection of impaired EGJ relaxation in a series of well defined achalasia patients. This is of great significance because failing to detect impaired EGJ relaxation has the result of giving these patients an alternative diagnosis, most commonly misclassifying as ineffective esophageal motility or DES.[4,13]

Apart from objectifying the definition of impaired deglutitive EGJ relaxation, EPT has also defined a clinically relevant subclassification of achalasia based on the

Table 1
Sensitivity of deglutitive EGJ relaxation measures in detecting achalasia

EGJ Relaxation Measure	Achalasia Sensitivity (%) (n = 62)	False Negative (%)
Single sensor nadir (<7 mm Hg)	52	48
High-resolution nadir (<10 mm Hg)	69	31
4-second integrated relaxation pressure (<15 mm Hg)	97	3

Data from Ghosh SK, Pandolfino JE, Rice J, et al. Impaired deglutitive EGJ relaxation in clinical esophageal manometry: a quantitative analysis of 400 patients and 75 controls. Am J Physiol Gastrointest Liver Physiol 2007;293(4):G878–85.

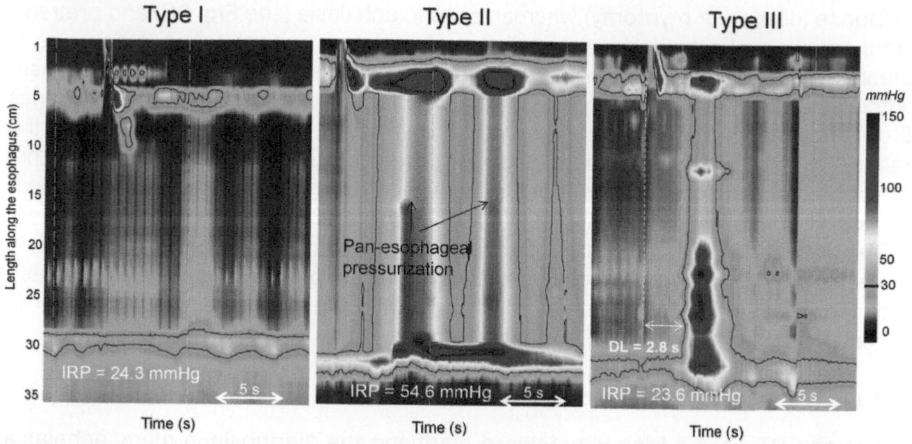

Fig. 3. Achalasia subtypes on esophageal pressure topography (EPT). Type I is characterized by an elevated integrated relaxation pressure (mean IRP >15 mm Hg) associated with absent contractile activity and negligible esophageal pressurization. Type II is characterized by an elevated IRP, absent contractile activity, and presence of pan-esophageal pressurization at 30 mm Hg IBC. Type III is characterized by elevated IRP and at least 20% of persistent contractions that are either incomplete or premature. In this example, the contraction is premature (DL <4.5 seconds).

pattern of "absent peristalsis" in the esophageal body.[14] Absent peristalsis is not synonymous with an absence of pressurization or contractile activity. Rather, absent peristalsis accompanying impaired EGJ relaxation can occur in the setting of esophageal dilatation with negligible pressurization within the esophagus (**Fig. 3**A), pan-esophageal pressurization (see **Fig. 3**B), or with some persistent contraction within the distal esophageal segment (see **Fig. 3**C). According to the Chicago Classification of EPT, the criteria for type I (classic) achalasia are an IRP of 15 mm Hg or greater and absent peristalsis; type II (achalasia with esophageal pressurization) has an IRP of 15 mm Hg or greater and at least 20% of swallows associated with panesophageal pressurization to greater than 30 mm Hg; and type III achalasia has an IRP of 15 mm Hg or greater and either a spastic contraction or a preserved peristaltic fragment with 20% or greater of test swallows.[14] Recent data suggest that classifying the etiology of the residual distal contraction in type III achalasia is best accomplished by measuring its latency relative to UES relaxation.[15] Premature contractions (latency <4.5 seconds) are indicative of spastic achalasia whereas normal latency contractions suggest a fragment of preserved peristalsis in the esophageal body. To add some perspective to the distribution of subtypes encountered, in a series of 99 consecutive patients with newly diagnosed achalasia, 21 had type I, 49 had type II, and 29 had type III.[14] Consequently, most of the patients in that series would not be diagnosed with achalasia according to a conventional manometric classification. The conventional diagnosis of "vigorous achalasia" (although it never had a precise definition) would likely include some cases of both type II and type III achalasia, diagnoses with nearly opposite implications, as detailed later.

The ultimate significance of identifying subtypes of achalasia is that it clarifies management, and preliminary data suggest this to be the case. Logistic regression analysis of predictors of treatment benefit in a large consecutive series found pan-esophageal pressurization (see **Fig. 3**B) to be a predictor of good treatment response (dilation or myotomy) whereas spastic achalasia (see **Fig. 3**C) and pretreatment esophageal dilatation were predictive of a relatively poor treatment response.[14] Clearly, these nuances have not been utilized in prior reports of achalasia treatment outcomes. Given that the mix of achalasia subtypes within any reported case series likely impacts on the efficacy observed in that series, this calls into question the validity of the existing treatment data in the era of EPT. It is our suspicion that adopting these subclassifications will likely strengthen the quality of future prospective studies of achalasia management, although this clearly requires further validation.

The impedance characteristics of achalasia are, as one would predict, incomplete bolus transit. Although that finding is supportive of the physiologic defect associated with the disease, it has not as yet been shown to help in subtyping achalasia or in assessing the effectiveness of a rendered therapy.

EGJ OUTFLOW OBSTRUCTION: IS IT ACHALASIA?

Although EPT goes a long way toward clarifying the diagnosis in many achalasia patients who would otherwise be classified as "nonspecific" or misclassified to a non-achalasia diagnosis, there is still a group of patients with impaired EGJ relaxation failing to meet criteria for achalasia because they demonstrate some preserved peristalsis. Though not common, a series of 1000 consecutive patients studied with EPT included 16 such individuals with EGJ outflow obstruction exhibiting not only an IRP greater than 15 mm Hg, but also preserved peristalsis and elevated intrabolus pressure above the EGJ during peristalsis.[16] The finding of elevated intrabolus pressure is important because it validates the determination of impaired EGJ relaxation. From a physiologic perspective, elevated intrabolus pressure is the consequence of that impaired relaxation. Nonetheless, EGJ outflow obstruction represents a heterogeneous group with some individuals having an incomplete expression of achalasia and others likely having an undetected mechanical cause of EGJ outflow obstruction such as hiatus hernia or esophageal stenosis. Consequently, it is a patient group that usually merits further intensive evaluation with imaging studies to exclude inflammatory or malignant etiologies, be that with computerized tomography or endoscopic ultrasound, before accepting it to be atypical achalasia.

Among the 16 patients with idiopathic EGJ outflow obstruction described in the preceding text, 3 were noted to have hiatus hernias. In one of these instances it was the crural diaphragm rather than the LES that appeared to be the focus of resistance to bolus transit, suggesting this be the cause of dysphagia. A subsequent report specifically focused on the EGJ relaxation characteristics of patients with sliding hiatus hernia and dysphagia by selectively restricting the IRP measurement boundaries to the LES and crural diaphragm individually.[17] A subset of 10 patients were found exhibiting a relative obstruction at the crural diaphragm with elevated intrabolus pressure extending through the LES, supporting the concept that sliding hiatus hernia could be responsible for dysphagia. Consequently, patients presenting with elevated EGJ relaxation pressure in the context of a small hiatus hernia require careful analysis of the discrete elements of the EGJ before a diagnosis of achalasia is made.

RETHINKING SPASM

Distal esophageal spasm (DES) is characterized by episodes of dysphagia and chest pain attributable to abnormal esophageal contractions in the setting of normal EGJ relaxation. Beyond that, there is little agreement. The pathophysiology and natural

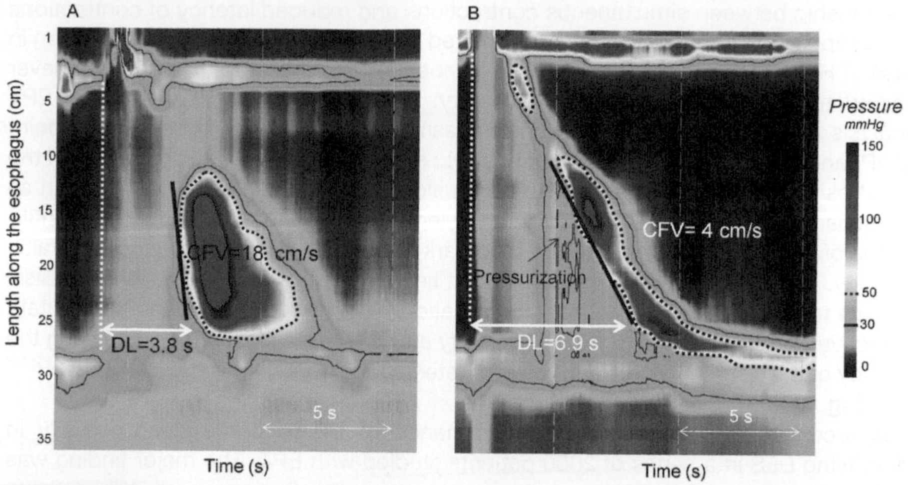

Fig. 4. Simultaneous contraction versus pressurization. The black line corresponds to 30 mm Hg IBC and the dashed one to 50 mm Hg IBC. Premature rapid contraction is represented in (*A*). DL and contractile front velocity (CFV) are measured at 30 mm Hg IBC. Note that 30 mm Hg and 50 mm Hg IBCs are parallel. The contraction in (*B*) is characterized by distal compartmentalized pressurization. The 30 mm Hg and 50 mm Hg IBCs are not parallel. DL and CFV are measured at 50 mm Hg to exclude the area of pressurization.

history of DES are ill defined. In radiologic publications, DES is commonly illustrated by tertiary contractions, a "corkscrew esophagus," or a "rosary bead esophagus," but in most instances these abnormalities are actually indicative of spastic achalasia. Manometrically, greatest consensus surrounds the concept of "simultaneous contractions" either with a defining minimum of 30 mm Hg or without defining amplitude.[18,19] By "simultaneous contractions" is meant that the upstroke of the pressure waves at adjacent recording sites (conventionally spaced 3–5 cm apart) occur at nearly the same instant. However, similar to the problems with the conventional manometric definition of achalasia, there is no distinction between pressure waves within the esophageal body attributable to intrabolus pressure or to contraction. Given these vagaries, it is likely that a heterogeneous group of patients have been diagnosed with DES and included in therapeutic trials of DES. Not surprisingly, none such studies have demonstrated efficacy.

Several nuances of defining DES emerge in EPT. First, there is a very important distinction to be made between a simultaneous contraction in the distal esophagus and simultaneous pressurization in the setting of EGJ outflow obstruction (**Fig. 4**). The former fits with the concept of DES whereas the latter is simply a consequence of impaired EGJ relaxation, most commonly in the setting of achalasia. Consequently, much of what would be labeled DES on the basis of "simultaneous contractions" in conventional manometry is actually achalasia.[4,14] Similarly, instances of "simultaneous contractions" of low amplitude are almost invariably attributable to intrabolus pressure in the setting of failed peristaltic contractions of subtle obstructive phenomenon in the distal esophagus.

An alternative metric for assessing propagation of peristalsis in EPT is the latency of the contraction in the distal esophagus. Behar and Biancani initially established the relationship between simultaneous contractions and reduced latency of contractions and proposed this to be indicative of impaired deglutitive inhibition, as can be seen in DES.[20] However, perhaps because it is cumbersome to measure, this concept never gained traction in conventional manometry. Two recently described tools in EPT analysis that improve the recognition of spasm are the contractile deceleration point (CDP) and the Distal Contractile Latency (DL; see **Fig. 1**). The CDP is the locus in the distal esophageal body characterized by a slowing of the deglutitive contraction as peristalsis terminates and ampullary emptying begins.[21] Consequently, the identification of the CDP provides a reliable landmark (the endpoint) for measuring peristaltic velocity. The DL is a related measure in that times the occurrence of distal peristalsis relative to deglutitive upper sphincter relaxation. Together, these measures facilitate objective measurement of peristaltic velocity and provide a means for quantifying the latency of the distal contraction as a surrogate for inhibitory ganglionic integrity[20,22,23] (see **Fig. 4**).

A recent study compared the performance of DL to propagation velocity in identifying DES in a series of 2000 patients studied with EPT. The major finding was that rapid contractile velocity was a very nonspecific finding, rarely the defining feature of a clinically significant disorder unless accompanied by reduced DL.[22] Tutuian and Castell similarly concluded that conventionally defined DES identified a very heterogeneous population based on an assessment of bolus transit in 33 such patients with combined manometry and impedance.[10] Reduced DL, however, was much better, both in terms of being a much less common and a much more homogeneous clinical entity. Affected patients almost uniformly had severe dysphagia. However, three quarters of these individuals were ultimately managed as an achalasia subtype (spastic achalasia), raising the question of whether or not spastic achalasia and "DES" are not actually minor variations on the same theme of impaired inhibitory neuronal function in the distal esophagus.

A much more consistent pattern of abnormal contractility in EPT is of very vigorous contractions with normal deglutitive EGJ relaxation and propagation velocity. In such instances, the distal esophageal contraction can be characterized for the vigor of contraction using a newly developed measure, the distal contractile integral (DCI). The DCI integrates the length, contractile amplitude, and duration of contraction of the distal esophageal segment contraction, expressed as mm Hg-s-cm.[24,25] Using data from control subjects, a mean DCI value greater than 5000 mm Hg-s-cm exceeds the 95th percentile of normal. This threshold is used in EPT analysis as the equivalent of "nutcracker esophagus" or "hypertensive peristalsis." Even more extreme is a patient group with a single swallow with DCI greater than 8000 mm Hg-s-cm, a magnitude never seen in normal subjects. These individuals are classified as having "hypercontractile esophagus" in EPT and are characterized by normal propagation velocity, DCI greater than 8000 mmHg-s-cm and no more than marginal abnormalities of the IRP. In many instances, the esophageal contraction is repetitive, earning it the nickname "jackhammer esophagus" in the latest iteration of the Chicago Classification of EPT.[26] Although the full clinical spectrum of these patients is not yet understood, essentially all are symptomatic with dysphagia or chest pain. From a physiologic perspective, the abnormality is of hyperexcitability of the distal esophageal smooth muscle, establishing a clear distinction from the impaired inhibitory innervation characteristic of achalasia and "DES." Consequently, given a plausible unifying pathophysiology, "hypercontractile" or "jackhammer" esophagus" is probably an appropriate target of future therapeutic trials.

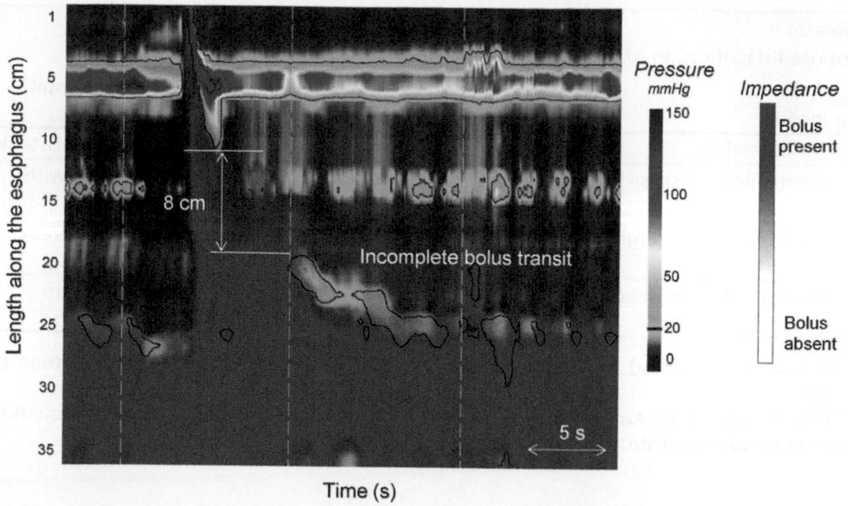

Fig. 5. High-resolution manometry combined with impedance. The black line represents the 20 mm Hg IBC. Impedance data are displayed by overlaid pink colorization, with the pink shading indicative of areas on the topography plots with retained bolus. The swallow is associated with a large proximal break (>5 cm) at 20 mm Hg IBC. The break is responsible of a bolus escape as attested by the persistence of the pink shadow.

WEAK PERISTALSIS

One of the major clinical applications of manometry is to assess the integrity of peristalsis, either as part of an evaluation of dysphagia or in anticipation of antireflux surgery. Conventionally, this is done by measuring the distal peristaltic amplitude.[18] The most commonly accepted metrics establishing normality are that peristaltic amplitude exceed 30 mm Hg at recording sites 3 and 8 cm proximal to the lower LES[18] based on the observation that amplitudes less than 30 mm Hg are frequently associated with bolus escape and incomplete bolus clearance on fluoroscopy.[27] However, with the evolution of intraluminal impedance monitoring and EPT it has become apparent that these conventional metrics provide a very incomplete assessment of peristaltic integrity. Findings from multichannel intraluminal impedance recordings suggest that the 30 mm Hg threshold value is too high in many instances[10] while EPT studies suggest that the arbitrary selection of two foci to measure pressure amplitude ignores much of the detail and variability inherent in the segmental architecture of the peristaltic contraction.[4]

The most comprehensive assessment of peristaltic integrity is achieved by combining the technologies of HRM and high-resolution intraluminal impedance monitoring. The combined study, called high-resolution impedance manometry or HRIM, depicts both EPT and bolus disposition on the same graphic (**Fig. 5**). HRIM data show that failed peristalsis is uniformly associated with incomplete bolus transit. With respect to hypotensive peristalsis, the critical finding in EPT is of breaks in the 20 or 30 mm Hg isobaric contour (IBC) delineating the peristaltic contraction spanning from the UES to the EGJ.[28,29] When 20 mm Hg IBC breaks exceed 5 cm in length, signifying that there is a 5 cm span of the esophagus with a peristaltic amplitude of less than 20 mm Hg, they are uniformly associated with incomplete bolus transit at that site gauged by the high-resolution impedance recording. When breaks are in the

Table 2
Proposed classification of peristaltic integrity in EPT

Diagnosis	Diagnostic Criteria (all with normal EGJ relaxation)
Absent peristalsis	100% of swallows with failed peristalsis
Frequent failed peristalsis[a]	>30%, but <100% of swallows with failed peristalsis
Weak peristalsis with large peristaltic defects	>20% of swallows with >5 cm breaks in the 20 mm Hg IBC
Weak peristalsis with small peristaltic defects	>30% of swallows with 2- to 5-cm breaks in the 20 mm Hg IBC

IBC pressure is referenced to atmospheric. Note that an individual may have more than one diagnosis.

[a] Although statistically exceeding the 95th percentile of normal, this finding has not been shown to correlate with nonobstructive dysphagia.

range of 2 to 5 cm they will variably be associated with incomplete bolus transit (IBT). Given these data, the frequency of occurrence of these three phenomena (failed peristalsis, large breaks in the 20 mm Hg IBC, and small breaks in the 20 mm Hg IBC) are indices of the adequacy of peristalsis for achieving esophageal bolus transit.

A recent study examined the relationship between these putative measures of weak peristalsis (failed peristalsis, larger breaks, and small breaks in the 20 mm Hg IBC) and nonobstructive dysphagia.[29] The major aims were to establish normal limits of peristaltic integrity in EPT terms based on a systematic analysis of a large series of control subjects, and to develop a classification scheme for weak peristalsis based on a comparison between control subjects and a cohort of patients with unexplained nonobstructive dysphagia intended for use in clinical EPT studies. The major findings were that the segmental architecture of peristalsis was highly stereotyped among subjects, as were defects in that architecture associated with incomplete bolus transit for individual subjects: large (>5 cm) and small (2–5 cm) breaks in the 20 mm Hg IBC of the peristaltic contraction. Although encountered in only about a third of the 113 patients studied, frequent large and small breaks in the 20 mm Hg IBC were significantly more common in the dysphagia patients than in control subjects. Failed peristalsis, the other mechanism of IBT observed in the HRIM studies, occurred no more frequently in the dysphagia population than in the control subjects. Based on these observations, an EPT classification of weak peristalsis has been proposed based on the occurrence of breaks in the 20 mm Hg IBC wherein weak peristalsis with large breaks is defined by these occurring with greater than 20% of swallows and weak peristalsis with small breaks defined by these occurring with grater than 30% of swallows (**Table 2**).

SUMMARY: THE EVOLVING CHICAGO CLASSIFICATION OF EPT

The preceding description of distal esophageal motility disorders in terms of EPT is a concise summation of an evolving process that has unfolded during the past 6 or 7 years as part of the International High Resolution Manometry Working Group. The evolving classification is referred to as the Chicago Classification and is being specifically developed to facilitate the interpretation of clinical EPT studies in clinical practice. The Chicago Classification has been, and will continue to be, an evolutionary process, molded first by published evidence and secondly by group experience when

Table 3
The Chicago Classification of esophageal motility

Diagnosis	Diagnostic Criteria
Achalasia	
Type I achalasia	Classic achalasia: mean IRP > upper limit of normal, 100% failed peristalsis
Type II achalasia	Achalasia with esophageal compression: mean IRP > upper limit of normal, no normal peristalsis, panesophageal pressurization with ≥20% of swallows
Type III achalasia	Mean IRP > upper limit of normal, no normal peristalsis, preserved fragments of distal peristalsis or premature (spastic) contractions with ≥20% of swallows
EGJ outflow obstruction	Mean IRP > upper limit of normal, some instances of intact peristalsis or weak peristalsis with small breaks such that the criteria for achalasia are not met[a]
Motility disorders	(patterns not observed in normal individuals)
Distal esophageal spasm	Normal mean IRP, ≥20% premature contractions
Hypercontractile (jackhammer) esophagus	At least one swallow DCI > 8000 mm Hg-s-cm with single peaked or multipeaked contraction[b]
Absent peristalsis	Normal mean IRP, 100% of swallows with failed peristalsis
Peristaltic abnormalities	*(defined by exceeding statistical limits of normal)*
Weak peristalsis with large peristaltic defects	Mean IRP <15 mm Hg and >20% swallows with large breaks in the 20 mm Hg IBC (>5 cm in length)
Weak peristalsis with small peristaltic defects	Mean IRP <15 mm Hg and >30% swallows with small breaks in the 20 mm Hg IBC (2–5 cm in length)
Frequent failed peristalsis	>30%, but <100% of swallows with failed peristalsis
Rapid contractions with normal latency	Rapid contraction with ≥20% of swallows, DL >4.5 seconds
Hypertensive peristalsis (nutcracker esophagus)	Mean DCI >5000 mmHg-s-cm, but not meeting criteria for hypercontractile esophagus
Normal	Not achieving any of the above diagnostic criteria

[a] May be a variant form of achalasia, indicative of wall stiffness consequent from an infiltrative disease, or manifestation of hiatal hernia in which case it can be subtyped to CD or LES.
[b] The locus of the multipeaked contraction can be in either of the distal two contractile segments or very rarely in the LES, but is usually this is in the third contractile segment. May coexist with EGJ outflow obstruction.

suitable evidence is lacking. The most recent iteration of his classification emerged from a meeting of the International High Resolution Manometry Working Group that occurred in Ascona, Switzerland in April, 2011 and is currently in the process of being published. The essential details of this are outlined in **Table 3**. Moving forward, we anticipate continuing this process with increased emphasis placed on natural history studies and outcome data based on the developing classification.

REFERENCES

1. Pandolfino JE, Kahrilas PJ. AGA technical review on the clinical use of esophageal manometry. Gastroenterology 2005;128(1):209–24.
2. Fox MR, Bredenoord AJ. Oesophageal high-resolution manometry: moving from research into clinical practice. Gut 2008;57(3):405–23.
3. Clouse RE, Staiano A, Alrakawi A. Development of a topographic analysis system for manometric studies in the gastrointestinal tract. Gastrointest Endosc 1998;48(4):395–401.
4. Clouse RE, Staiano A, Alrakawi A, et al. Application of topographical methods to clinical esophageal manometry. Am J Gastroenterol 2000;95(10):2720–30.
5. Silny J. Intraluminal multiple electrical impedance procedure for measurement of gastrointestinal motility. J Gastroenterol Motil 1991;3:151–62.
6. Sifrim D, Silny J, Holloway RH, et al. Patterns of gas and liquid reflux during transient lower oesophageal sphincter relaxation: a study using intraluminal electrical impedance. Gut 1999;44(1):47–54.
7. Silny J, Knigge KP, Fass J, et al. Verification of the intraluminal multiple electrical impedance measurement for the recording of gastrointestinal motility. J Gastrointest Motil 1993;5:107–22.
8. Kahrilas PJ. Will impedence testing rewrite the book on GERD? Gastroenterology 2001;120(7):1862–4.
9. Tutuian R, Vela MF, Balaji NS, et al. Esophageal function testing with combined multichannel intraluminal impedance and manometry: multicenter study in healthy volunteers. Clin Gastroenterol Hepatol 2003;1(3):174–82.
10. Tutuian R, Castell DO. Combined multichannel intraluminal impedance and manometry clarifies esophageal function abnormalities: study in 350 patients. Am J Gastroenterol 2004;99(6):1011–9.
11. Pandolfino JE, Kahrilas PJ, American Gastroenterological Association. American Gastroenterological Association medical position statement: clinical use of esophageal manometry. Gastroenterology 2005;128(1):207–8.
12. Ghosh SK, Pandolfino JE, Rice J, et al. Impaired deglutitive EGJ relaxation in clinical esophageal manometry: a quantitative analysis of 400 patients and 75 controls. Am J Physiol Gastrointest Liver Physiol 2007;293(4):G878–85.
13. Fox M, Hebbard G, Janiak P, et al. High-resolution manometry predicts the success of oesophageal bolus transport and identifies clinically important abnormalities not detected by conventional manometry. Neurogastroenterol Motil 2004;16(5):533–42.
14. Pandolfino JE, Kwiatek MA, Nealis T, et al. Achalasia: a new clinically relevant classification by high-resolution manometry. Gastroenterology 2008;135(5):1526–33.
15. McCarthy ST, Cluley JD, Roman S, et al. Spastic achalasia phenotypes in esophageal pressure topography (EPT): not all spasm is the same. Gastroenterology 2011;140(5[Suppl 1]):S-77.
16. Scherer JR, Kwiatek MA, Soper NJ, et al. Functional esophagogastric junction obstruction with intact peristalsis: a heterogeneous syndrome sometimes akin to achalasia. J Gastrointest Surg 2009;13(12):2219–25.
17. Pandolfino JE, Kwiatek MA, Ho K, et al. Unique features of esophagogastric junction pressure topography in hiatus hernia patients with dysphagia. Surgery 2010;147(1):57–64.
18. Spechler SJ, Castell DO. Classification of oesophageal motility abnormalities. Gut 2001;49(1):145–51.

19. Dalton CB, Castell DO, Hewson EG, et al. Diffuse esophageal spasm. A rare motility disorder not characterized by high-amplitude contractions. Dig Dis Sci 1991;36(8): 1025–8.
20. Behar J, Biancani P. Pathogenesis of simultaneous esophageal contractions in patients with motility disorders. Gastroenterology 1993;105(1):111–8.
21. Pandolfino JE, Leslie E, Luger D, et al. The contractile deceleration point: an important physiologic landmark on oesophageal pressure topography. Neurogastroenterol Motil 2010;22(4):395–400.
22. Pandolfino JE, Roman S, Carlson D, et al. Distal esophageal spasm in high resolution esophageal pressure topography: defining clinical phenotypes. Gastroenterology 2011;141(2):469–75.
23. Roman S, Lin Z, Pandolfino JE, et al. Distal contraction latency: a measure of propagation velocity optimized for esophageal pressure topography studies. Am J Gastroenterol 2011;106(3):443–51.
24. Ghosh SK, Pandolfino JE, Zhang Q, et al. Quantifying esophageal peristalsis with high-resolution manometry: a study of 75 asymptomatic volunteers. Am J Physiol Gastrointest Liver Physiol 2006;290(5):G988–997.
25. Pandolfino JE, Ghosh SK, Rice J, et al. Classifying esophageal motility by pressure topography characteristics: a study of 400 patients and 75 controls. Am J Gastroenterol 2008;103(1):27–37.
26. Roman S, Pandolfino JE, Chen J, et al. Phenotypes and clinical context of hypercontractility in high-resolution esophageal pressure topography (EPT). Am J Gastroenterol 2011. [Epub ahead of print].
27. Kahrilas PJ, Dodds WJ, Hogan WJ. Effect of peristaltic dysfunction on esophageal volume clearance. Gastroenterology 1988;94(1):73–80.
28. Bulsiewicz WJ, Kahrilas PJ, Kwiatek MA, et al. Esophageal pressure topography criteria indicative of incomplete bolus clearance: a study using high-resolution impedance manometry. Am J Gastroenterol 2009;104(11):2721–8.
29. Roman S, Lin Z, Kwiatek MA, et al. Weak peristalsis in esophageal pressure topography: classification and association with dysphagia. Am J Gastroenterol 2011; 106(2):349–56.

Difficult Defecation: Difficult Problem Assessment and Management; What Really Helps?

Adil E. Bharucha, MBBS, MD

KEYWORDS

• Defecatory disorders • Defecation • Pelvic floor dysfunction
• Puborectalis • Anorectal • Biofeedback

A subset of patients with chronic constipation, up to 50% at tertiary centers, have difficult defecation, which can be suspected by clinical features and confirmed by anorectal tests. Symptoms of difficult defecation (ie, defecatory disorders) may occur in isolation or in association with symptoms of irritable bowel syndrome. Patients with defecatory disorders may have normal or slow colonic transit. Defecatory disorders should be recognized early because pelvic floor retraining by biofeedback therapy is superior to laxatives for management.

CLINICAL FEATURES

Among people with chronic constipation, clinical experience suggests that some symptoms, such as the excessive straining or the sense of anorectal obstruction/blockage during defecation and the use of manual maneuvers (ie, vaginal splinting or anal digitation) to facilitate defecation are suggestive of defecatory disorders.[1,2] Other symptoms (eg, lumpy or hard stools, sensation of incomplete evacuation, less than3 defecations/week) are not. Moreover, symptoms should be interpreted in the context of stool consistency, which should be preferably characterized by asking patients to refer to a Bristol stool form scale.[3] While normal people may experience difficulty in evacuating hard stools, difficulty in evacuating soft stools or enema fluid is particularly

This project was supported by USPHS NIH Grant R01 DK78924. The author has nothing to disclose.
Clinical Enteric Neurosciences Translational and Epidemiological Research Program, Division of Gastroenterology and Hepatology, Mayo Clinic and Mayo Foundation, 200 1st Street SW, Rochester, MN 55905, USA
E-mail address: bharucha.adil@mayo.edu

Gastroenterol Clin N Am 40 (2011) 837–844
doi:10.1016/j.gtc.2011.09.001
0889-8553/11/$ – see front matter

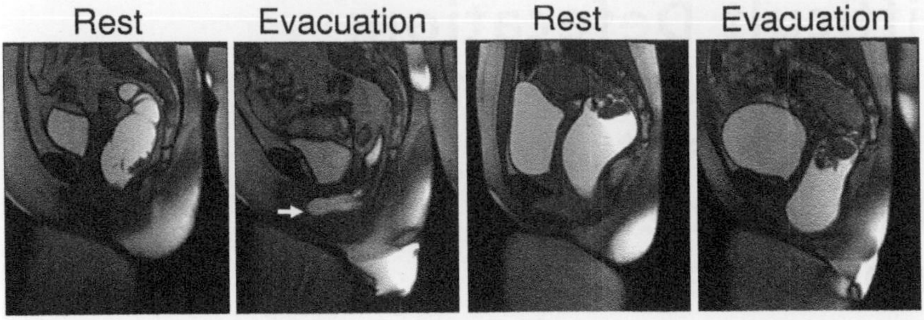

Fig. 1. Magnetic resonance fluoroscopic images of the pelvis in two patients with symptoms of difficult defecation. The rectum was filled with ultrasound gel. Observe normal perineal descent, pelvic floor relaxation, normal rectal evacuation with a 3.8 cm anterior rectocele (*white arrow*), which incompletely empties in the left panel. In the right panel, despite normal perineal descent, indicative of straining, the anal canal did not open and rectal evacuation was incomplete.

suggestive of defecatory disorders. Not infrequently, irritable bowel syndrome and pelvic floor dysfunction will coexist.[4]

In defecatory disorders, inspection of the anal orifice may reveal anal fissures or large hemorrhoids in patients with pelvic floor dysfunction. Digital rectal examination can assess anal pressure at rest, when patients contract or squeeze their anal sphincter and pelvic floor muscles, and during simulated evacuation.[5] Normally, simulated evacuation is accompanied by relaxation of the anal sphincter and puborectalis muscle and perineal descent by 1 to 4 cm (**Fig. 1**). Patients with defecatory disorders have one or more abnormal findings, including anismus (ie, high anal resting pressure), reduced or excessive perineal descent (ie, ballooning of the perineum), and/or rectal prolapse. The puborectalis may not relax normally or, paradoxically, may contract during simulated evacuation. In my experience, relaxation of the puborectalis may not be perceptible even in patients with normal anorectal functions. Therefore, except for patients who have paradoxical puborectalis contraction, abnormal perineal descent, particularly if markedly reduced or absent, is more useful than impaired puborectalis relaxation for identifying defecatory disorders. Similar to anorectal testing, the digital rectal examination is influenced, to a greater extent in some patients than others, by the vagaries of trying to simulate defecation in the left lateral position in a physician's office.

Nonetheless, 2 recent studies observed that a careful digital examination compared favorably to objective assessments of anorectal functions.[6–8] In the first study, there was excellent agreement, as evidenced by a correlation coefficient of 0.8, between anal resting and squeeze pressures graded by the digital rectal examination scoring system (DRESS) and anorectal manometry in 383 patients with defecatory symptoms of whom 303 patients had a complete data set.[6] In another cohort of 209 patients (191 men) with symptoms of chronic constipation, 134 of 183 patients (73%) with dyssynergia by anorectal manometry also had dyssynergia on a digital rectal examination (ie, "digital dyssynergia").[7] Digital dyssynergia was identified on the basis of the presence of 2 or more of the following features: impaired perineal descent, paradoxical anal contraction, or impaired push effort. Four patients, however, who had "digital dyssynergia" had normal manometry. Hence, a digital rectal examination was 75% sensitive and 87% specific for diagnosing dyssynergia as predicted by manometry; the corresponding positive and negative predictive values were 97% and 37%, respectively. Among 94 patients who had an abnormal balloon expulsion test, which is the most sensitive and specific test for diagnosing rectal evacuation disorder,[9] 75 (80%) of patients had digital dyssynergia. But 59 of 115 patients (51%) with a normal balloon expulsion test also had "digital dyssynergia"; hence a digital exam was 56% specific relative to rectal balloon expulsion. While there was good agreement (>85%) between the digital rectal examination and manometry for identifying a normal anal resting and squeeze pressures, agreement for identifying weak resting and squeeze pressures was fair (approximately 50% to 55%). In summary, a digital rectal examination is useful for assessing anal functions, should be interpreted in the context of symptoms, and when necessary, particularly in patients with suspected defecatory disorders, confirmed by anorectal manometry. In chronic constipation, a normal test is more useful than an abnormal test.

ANORECTAL TESTS

Anorectal tests should be performed in constipated patients who do not respond to simple laxatives, or even earlier, in patients who have symptoms and signs of difficult defecation. In most patients, anorectal manometry and a rectal balloon expulsion test suffice to confirm or exclude defecatory disorders. In selected circumstances (ie, when only one test is abnormal, when pelvic organ prolapse or a large rectocoele is suspected, or when there is a discrepancy between the clinical features and these anorectal tests), barium or magnetic resonance (MR) defecography is necessary to break the tie.[10,11]

The rectal balloon expulsion test is a very simple, sensitive, and specific test for diagnosing defecatory disorders.[9] Patients are asked to expel a 4-cm rectal balloon filled with 50 ml of warm water while seated on a commode; normally this requires less than 1 minute; patients with defecatory disorders require more time or cannot expel the balloon.[12] Alternatively, patients are asked to expel a rectal balloon, connected over a pulley to weights, in the left lateral decubitus position; patients with pelvic floor dysfunction require more external traction to expel the balloon.[10] Perception of the desire to defecate is essential prior to normal defecation. Some patients with defecatory disorders have reduced rectal sensation.[13] While most laboratories inflate a rectal balloon by a standard volume, typically 50 ml, it has been suggested that when rectal sensation is reduced, patients may not perceive the desire to defecate at a volume of 50 ml, limiting their ability to evacuate the balloon even though rectal evacuation is preserved.[9] An alternative approach is to inflate the balloon by increasing volumes until patients experience the desire to defecate.[9] These 2 techniques (ie, fixed versus variable balloon inflation) of assessing rectal evacuation have not been compared in patients.

Anal manometry may reveal a high anal resting pressure or anismus (ie, 90 mm Hg or greater) in defecatory disorders. [11]A reduced rectoanal pressure gradient, expressed as the ratio or the difference between rectal and anal pressure, during simulated evacuation, is also used to identify disordered rectal evacuation.[14] However, in my experience, this measure is not as useful as a balloon expulsion test since (1) dyssynergia did not predict an abnormal rectal balloon expulsion test in healthy people,[15] (2) many asymptomatic people also have an "abnormal" gradient during simulated evacuation,[16] and (3) there is considerable overlap in the rectoanal pressure gradient between health and defecatory disorders and, among constipated patients, between patients who have and do not have a defecatory disorder.[17] Hence, further studies to evaluate the utility of the rectoanal pressure gradient for identifying defecatory disorders are necessary. Except for Hirschsprung's disease, the rectoanal inhibitory reflex is preserved in chronic constipation.

Barium or MR defecography can identify structural abnormalities (eg, rectocele, enterocele, and rectal prolapse) and evaluate anorectal motion by measuring various parameters (ie, anorectal angle, perineal descent, anal diameter, puborectalis indentation and rectal contents) at rest, during voluntary contraction, and during rectal evacuation.[18] Barium defecography should be performed with barium paste rather than liquid barium and radiologists should be encouraged to measure anorectal parameters in addition to providing an overall impression. It can be challenging to measure these parameters because the bony landmarks necessary for making these measurements may not be clearly visible. Hence, perineal descent is measured relative to markings on a commode. MR defecography overcomes this limitation and, in contrast to barium defecography, does not entail radiation exposure, and also visualizes bladder and urogenital prolapse. In a controlled study, MR defecography identified disturbances of evacuation and/or squeeze in 94% of patients with suspected defecation disorders.[10] In addition to examining the images, I also find it useful to review real-time images of the defecography.

While these anorectal tests are useful for identifying defecatory disorders, there are several caveats to interpreting test results. First, these tests may be abnormal even in asymptomatic people.[19,20] Second, the literature suggests there is a relatively poor correlation among various tests (eg, anorectal manometry and defecography) in patients with defecatory disorders and that there is no true gold standard diagnostic test. Third, it is my perception that some patients with clinical features of pelvic floor dysfunction have seemingly normal rectal evacuation by testing, perhaps because they strain excessively to overcome increased pelvic floor resistance. Thus, an integrated assessment of clinical features and anorectal tests is necessary to confirm or exclude defecation disorders.

MANAGEMENT

Pelvic Floor Retraining by Biofeedback Therapy

Pelvic floor retraining by biofeedback therapy, supplemented by laxatives if necessary to ensure soft stools, improves symptoms in a majority of patients with defecatory disorders. Patients are educated about the normal physiology of defecation; errors in their process are identified. Using electronically augmented feedback, patients learn how to relax or contract muscles at appropriate times and to strain appropriately (ie, increase intra-abdominal pressure) while ensuring that pelvic floor muscles, as evidenced by EMG activity or anal canal pressures, are relaxed. Subsequently, patients learn how to evacuate an air-filled balloon while therapists assist by pulling on a catheter attached to the balloon. Some centers also include sensory training to teach the patient how to recognize weaker sensations of rectal filling. At Mayo Clinic, we provide 2 or 3 sessions daily over 2 weeks, primarily for patient convenience. Other centers provide 5 or 6 biweekly sessions lasting 30 to 60 minutes. Controlled studies show that pelvic floor retraining is superior to laxatives alone,[21] to sham treatment (relaxation therapy),[22] or to diazepam or placebo[23] for improving symptoms and anorectal functions in defecatory disorders. This improvement is sustained at 12 and 24 months.[21,24] An abnormal rectal balloon expulsion test predicts the response to biofeedback therapy.[25]

There are several logistical challenges to providing biofeedback therapy for defecatory disorders. In the United States, for example, many insurance programs do not cover pelvic floor retraining by biofeedback therapy for chronic constipation but the situation is improving. While many therapists are familiar with Kegel's exercises, biofeedback therapy for defecatory disorders is not widely available.

Therapeutic options for patients who do not respond to biofeedback therapy are limited and unsatisfactory. Some patients with medically-refractory constipation after pelvic floor function normalizes have colonic motor dysfunction, as evidenced by delayed colonic transit and, if available, colonic intraluminal assessments (ie, by manometry and/or a barostat).[26] A subtotal colectomy with ileorectal anastomosis should be considered in these patients provided pelvic floor functions are normal. In general, poorer outcomes, in terms of satisfaction, are reported by authors who did not perform complete physiologic assessments of their patients; patients with delayed colonic transit and no pelvic floor dysfunction report higher rates of satisfaction and better function[27–29] than those who were operated upon based on history and physical exams alone.[30,31]

Pelvic Floor Botulinum Toxin Injection

Uncontrolled studies suggest that injection of botulinum toxin into the puborectalis muscle improves symptoms and anorectal functions in some patients with defecatory disorders.[32] The evidence that botulinum toxin is effective for defecatory disorders is inconclusive. Consistent with the mechanisms of action of botulinum toxin, the effects, when observed, are relatively brief. I have not found this approach useful in a small number of patients with defecatory disorders refractory to biofeedback therapy in which it has been tried.

Sacral Nerve Stimulation

There are some studies of sacral nerve stimulation (SNS) to treat the symptoms of constipation (caused by slow transit, pelvic floor dysfunction, or both) from Europe. In the largest, and a multicenter study, 45 of 62 patients with medically-refractory chronic constipation proceeded to permanent stimulation; 39 patients had improved symptoms (ie, 50% or greater reduction in straining during defecation, or sense of incomplete evacuation after defecation or an increase in bowel frequency from less than 3 to 3 or more bowel movements per week).[33] Of 27 patients in whom colonic transit was evaluated at baseline, 20 had delayed colonic transit; only 9 had delayed transit after therapy.[33] In contrast, another study of 19 patients reported only 42% of a mix of slow transit and pelvic floor patients improved with SNS.[34] Moreover, about 60% of patients receiving SNS for constipation experienced one or more "events"; the 2 most common were loss of efficacy and pain.[35] More than one-third of patients required surgical reintervention or discontinuation of treatment altogether.[35] SNS for constipation is not FDA approved for use in the United States.

Surgery for Rectocele and Rectal Intussusception

Small rectoceles are common in older women. Rectoceles, which are large (greater than 4 cm diameter), symptomatic (ie, require rectal splinting during defecation), and/or empty incompletely during defecation, are more likely to be clinically significant.[36,37] Perhaps rectocoeles may reflect "give-way" of the anterior rectal wall, often in the context of deficient support mechanisms (eg, after a hysterectomy). It is important to recognize that rectocoeles are often secondary rather than primary abnormalities; that is, they may be caused by excessive straining in patients with impaired pelvic floor relaxation. Hence pelvic floor retraining should initially be considered for managing rectoceles and rectal intussusception; surgical approaches to manage the latter are ineffective.[38,39] Impaired emptying of a rectocele may contribute not only to symptoms of disordered defecation but also to "passive" leakage (ie, after defecation) in fecal incontinence.

Stapled transanal resection (STARR) was developed to address the problem of obstructed defecation caused by 2 anatomic abnormalities: rectal intussusception (occult rectal prolapse) and rectoceles. This procedure staples the redundant rectal mucosa associated with rectocele and intussusception. The objective is to cure symptoms by resecting redundant tissue. However, the link between symptoms and actual anatomic abnormalities is tenuous.[40] It is probable that anatomic abnormalities (ie, intussusception and complete rectal prolapse) are caused by impaired pelvic floor relaxation and excessive straining, which is not corrected by the procedure. While a large randomized prospective multicenter trial observed that STARR was superior to pelvic floor retraining using biofeedback therapy, it is unclear what proportion of patients had pelvic floor dysfunction at baseline since rectal balloon expulsion was not evaluated at baseline; anal pressures were measured but not provided.[41] The effects on symptoms and anatomy were not correlated.[42–45] Complications include pelvic sepsis, fistula, peritonitis, bowel perforation, pain, and bleeding,[43,46,47] which has prompted pleas that only qualified surgeons perform STARR.[47] The long-term outcomes of patients, even when ideally suited for STARR, are disappointing.[48] The operation has failed to gain widespread acceptance in the United States.

Pouch of Douglas protrusion,[49] which is often confused with rectal intussusception and full-thickness rectal prolapse, is best addressed with sacrocolpopexy and is usually performed in conjunction with other gynecologic procedures in patients with pelvic floor abnormalities such as cystoceles, rectoceles, enteroceles, and vaginal vault prolapsed.[50]

Partial division of the puborectalis or anal sphincters can result in fecal incontinence and should not be considered for a functional disorder. Hence, a diverting ileostomy is perhaps the preferred option for patients with refractory pelvic floor dysfunction.

SUMMARY

Difficult defecation is a common and perhaps underrecognized cause of chronic constipation. While the history and a careful digital rectal examination are very useful for diagnosing defecatory disorders, the diagnosis needs to be confirmed by anorectal tests. Anorectal manometry and a rectal balloon expulsion test generally suffice to diagnose defecatory disorders; barium or MR defecography may necessary in selected cases. Colonic transit is normal or slow in patients with defecatory disorders. Pelvic floor retraining by biofeedback therapy is superior to laxatives for managing defecatory disorders.

REFERENCES

1. Koch A, Voderholzer WA, Klauser AG, et al. Symptoms in chronic constipation. Dis Colon Rectum 1997;40:902–6.
2. Bharucha AE, Wald A, Enck P, et al. Functional anorectal disorders. Gastroenterology 2006;130:1510–8.
3. Bharucha AE, Seide BM, Zinsmeister AR, et al. Insights into normal and disordered bowel habits from bowel diaries. Am J Gastroenterol 2008;103:692–8.
4. Suttor VP, Prott GM, Hansen RD, et al. Evidence for pelvic floor dyssynergia in patients with irritable bowel syndrome. Dis Colon Rectum 2010;53:156–60.
5. Jiang X, Locke GR 3rd, Choung RS, et al. Prevalence and risk factors for abdominal bloating and visible distention: a population-based study. Gut 2008;57:756–63.
6. Orkin BA, Sinykin SB, Lloyd PC. The digital rectal examination scoring system (DRESS). Dis Colon Rectum 2010;53(12):1656–60.
7. Tantiphlachiva K, Rao P, Attaluri A, et al. Digital rectal examination is a useful tool for identifying patients with dyssynergia. Clin Gastroenterol Hepatol 2010;8(11):955–60.
8. Bharucha AE. Recent advances in functional anorectal disorders. Curr Gastroenterol Rep 2011;13:316–22.

9. Minguez M, Herreros B, Sanchiz V, et al. Predictive value of the balloon expulsion test for excluding the diagnosis of pelvic floor dyssynergia in constipation. Gastroenterology 2004;126:57–62.
10. Bharucha AE, Fletcher JG, Seide B, et al. Phenotypic variation in functional disorders of defecation. Gastroenterology 2005;128:1199–210.
11. Fletcher JG, Busse RF, Riederer SJ, et al. Magnetic resonance imaging of anatomic and dynamic defects of the pelvic floor in defecatory disorders. Am J Gastroenterol. 2003 Feb;98:399–411.
12. Rao SS, Hatfield R, Soffer E, et al. Manometric tests of anorectal function in healthy adults. Am J Gastroenterol 1999;94:773–83.
13. Gladman MA, Lunniss PJ, Scott SM, et al. Rectal hyposensitivity. American Journal of Gastroenterology 2006;101:1140–51.
14. Rao SS, Welcher KD, Leistikow JS. Obstructive defecation: a failure of rectoanal coordination. Am J Gastroenterol 1998;93:1042–50.
15. Rao SSC, Kavlock R, Rao S. Influence of body position and stool characteristics on defecation in humans. Am J Gastroenterol 2006;101:2790–6.
16. Ravi K, Zinsmeister AR, Bharucha AE. Do rectoanal pressures predict rectal balloon expulsion in chronic constipation?. Gastroenterology 2009;136:A101–2.
17. Rao SS, Welcher KD, Leistikow JS. Obstructive defecation: a failure of rectoanal coordination. Am J Gastroenterol 1998;93:1042–50.
18. Barnett JL, Hasler WE, Camilleri M. American Gastroenterological Association medical position statement on anorectal testing techniques. Gastroenterology 1999;116:732–60.
19. Freimanis MG, Wald A, Caruana B, et al. Evacuation proctography in normal volunteers. Investig Radiol 1991;26:581–5.
20. Voderholzer WA, Neuhaus DA, Klauser AG, et al. Paradoxical sphincter contraction is rarely indicative of anismus. Gut 1997;41:258–62.
21. Chiarioni G, Whitehead WE, Pezza V, et al. Biofeedback is superior to laxatives for normal transit constipation due to pelvic floor dyssynergia. Gastroenterology 2006; 130:657–64.
22. Rao SS, Seaton K, Miller M, et al. Randomized controlled trial of biofeedback, sham feedback, and standard therapy for dyssynergic defecation. Clin Gastroenterol Hepatol 2007;5:331–8.
23. Heymen S, Scarlett Y, Jones K, et al. Randomized controlled trial shows biofeedback to be superior to alternative treatments for fecal incontinence. Dis Colon Rectum 2009;52:1730–7.
24. Rao SSC, Valestin J, Brown CK, et al. Long-term efficacy of biofeedback therapy for dyssynergic defecation: randomized controlled trial. Am J Gastroenterol 2010;105:890–6.
25. Chiarioni G, Salandini L, Whitehead WE. Biofeedback benefits only patients with outlet dysfunction, not patients with isolated slow transit constipation. Gastroenterology 2005;129:86–97.
26. Ravi K, Bharucha AE, Camilleri M, et al. Phenotypic Variation of colonic motor functions in chronic constipation. Gastroenterology 2009;138:89–97.
27. Pemberton JH, Rath DM, Ilstrup DM. Evaluation and surgical treatment of severe chronic constipation. Ann Surg 1991;214:403–11; discussion 411–3.
28. Nyam DC, Pemberton JH, Ilstrup DM, et al. Long-term results of surgery for chronic constipation. [Erratum appears in Dis Colon Rectum 1997 May;40:529]. Dis Colon Rectum 1997;40:273–9.
29. You YT, Wang JY, Changchien CR, et al. Segmental colectomy in the management of colonic inertia. Am Surg 1998;64:775–7.
30. Kamm MA, Hawley PR, Lennard-Jones JE. Outcome of colectomy for severe idiopathic constipation. Gut 1988;29:969–73.

31. Kuijpers HC. Application of the colorectal laboratory in diagnosis and treatment of functional constipation. Dis Colon Rectum 1990;33:35–9.
32. Maria G, Cadeddu F, Brandara F, et al. Experience with type A botulinum toxin for treatment of outlet-type constipation. Am J Gastroenterol 2006;101(11):2570–5.
33. Kamm MA, Dudding TC, Melenhorst J, et al. Sacral nerve stimulation for intractable constipation. Gut 2010;59:333–40.
34. Holzer B, Rosen HR, Novi G, et al. Sacral nerve stimulation in patients with severe constipation. Dis Colon Rectum 2008;51:524–9; discussion 529–30.
35. Maeda Y, Lundby L, Buntzen S, et al. Sacral nerve stimulation for constipation: suboptimal outcome and adverse events. Dis Colon Rectum 2010;53:995–9.
36. Kelvin FM, Maglinte DD, Hale DS, et al. Female pelvic organ prolapse: a comparison of triphasic dynamic MR imaging and triphasic fluoroscopic cystocolpoproctography. Am J Roentgenol 2000;174:81–8.
37. Ellerkmann RM, Cundiff GW, Melick CF, et al. Correlation of symptoms with location and severity of pelvic organ prolapse. Am J Obstet Gynecol 2001;185:1332–7; discussion 1337–8.
38. Orrom WJ, Bartolo DC, Miller R, et al. Rectopexy is an ineffective treatment for obstructed defecation. Dis Colon Rectum 1991;34:41–6.
39. Graf W, Karlbom U, Pahlman L, et al. Functional results after abdominal suture rectopexy for rectal prolapse or intussusception. Eur J Surg 1996;162(11):905–11.
40. Farouk R, Bhardwaj R, Phillips RKS. Stapled transanal resection of the rectum (STARR) for the obstructed defaecation syndrome. Ann R Coll Surg Engl 2009;91:287–91.
41. Lehur PA, Stuto A, Fantoli M, et al. Outcomes of stapled transanal rectal resection vs. biofeedback for the treatment of outlet obstruction associated with rectal intussusception and rectocele: a multicenter, randomized, controlled trial.[Erratum appears in Dis Colon Rectum. 2008 Nov;51:1739 Note: Narisetty, Prashanty (corrected to Narisetty, Prashanthi)]. Dis Colon Rectum 2008;51(11):1611–8.
42. Reboa G, Gipponi M, Logorio M, et al. The impact of stapled transanal rectal resection on anorectal function in patients with obstructed defecation syndrome. Dis Colon Rectum 2009;52:1598–604.
43. Titu LV, Riyad K, Carter H, et al. Stapled transanal rectal resection for obstructed defecation: a cautionary tale. Dis Colon Rectum 2009;52(10):1716–22.
44. Gagliardi G, Pescatori M, Altomare DF, et al. Results, outcome predictors, and complications after stapled transanal rectal resection for obstructed defecation. Dis Colon Rectum 2008;51:186–95; discussion 195.
45. Schwandner T, Hecker A, Hirschburger M, et al. Does the STARR procedure change the pelvic floor: a preoperative and postoperative study with dynamic pelvic floor MRI. Dis Colon Rectum 2011;54:412–7.
46. Dodi G, Pietroletti R, Milito G, et al. Bleeding, incontinence, pain and constipation after STARR transanal double stapling rectotomy for obstructed defecation. Techn Coloproctol 2003;7:148-3.
47. Corman ML, Carriero A, Hager T, et al. Consensus conference on the stapled transanal rectal resection (STARR) for disordered defaecation. Colorectal Dis 2006;8:98–101.
48. Madbouly KM, Abbas KS, Hussein AM. Disappointing long-term outcomes after stapled transanal rectal resection for obstructed defecation. World J Surg 2010;34:2191–6.
49. Jorge JM, Yang YK, Wexner SD. Incidence and clinical significance of sigmoidoceles as determined by a new classification system. Dis Colon Rectum 1994;37(11):1112–7.
50. Maher C, Feiner B, Baessler K, et al. Surgical management of pelvic organ prolapse in women. Cochrane Database Syst Rev 2010;4:CD004014.

Nutritional Support in the Severely Compromised Motility Patient: When and How?

Francisca Joly, MD, PhD*, Aurelien Amiot, MD,
Bernard Messing, MD, PhD

KEYWORDS

- Chronic intestinal pseudo-obstruction
- Home parenteral nutrition • Parenteral nutrition
- Compromised motility

Chronic intestinal pseudo-obstruction (CIPO) is today a significant indication for home parenteral nutrition (HPN) in both adults and children. CIPO refers to a heterogeneous group of disorders characterized by symptoms of intestinal obstruction in the absence of mechanical evidence of obstruction. It is caused by ineffective intestinal contractions. CIPO may be classified either as a primary disease, which is usually limited to the hollow viscera, or as a secondary disease, which is associated with an existing systemic disorder. CIPO may predominate as a "total" gut disease from esophagus to anal sphincter or as a "localized" disease, which is gastric and intestinal or intestinal alone; with the exception of an isolated megaduodenum, segmental gut disease is not a feature. Recurrent episodes of obstruction are the usual clinical presentation with, most frequently, malabsorptive diarrhea; pseudo-pseudo CIPO may also be a manifestation, ie, malabsorptive diarrhea without obvious obstruction. Besides nutritional support, symptomatic treatment usually consists of prokinetic drugs, such as low-dose octreotide or erythromycin. In the case of a systemic disease causing CIPO, specific treatment directed against the primary disease process is another cornerstone of management, for example, in systemic lupus erythematosus. The most severe forms may require ostomies for provision of nutrition or decompression. Other surgical interventions are best avoided, with the exception of those required for such complications of CIPO as peritonitis caused by perforation (with or without diverticula) or bowel ischemia. Patients with the most severe forms of CIPO and, especially, those affected by the diffuse forms of the disease, and who have, in

Department of Gastroenterology and Nutrition Support, Beaujon Hospital, René Diderot University of Paris, 100 bd Général Leclerc 92100, Clichy, France
* Corresponding author.
E-mail address: francisca.joly@bjn.aphp.fr

Gastroenterol Clin N Am 40 (2011) 845–851
doi:10.1016/j.gtc.2011.09.010 gastro.theclinics.com
0889-8553/11/$ – see front matter

effect, a "functional" intestinal failure, may need long-term HPN. In the latter case, when there is a failure of HPN, alternative treatments, such as extensive resection or intestinal transplantation, should be discussed on a case-by-case basis in a intestinal tertiary care center.

EPIDEMIOLOGY

The heterogeneity of the disease and the lack of large-scale observational studies contribute to the absence of good epidemiologic data on CIPO. Based on the registry of the American Pseudo-Obstruction and Hirschsprung's Society (now part of the International Foundation for Functional Gastrointestinal Disorders), the incidence of the neonatal form of CIPO in the United States has been estimated at 100 per year (equivalent to 0.3 pediatric cases per million births per year).[1] The French Web registry of Home Parenteral Nutrition (HPN) collects data on patients with intestinal failure requiring HPN: in this database, CIPO comprises 10% of all adult and infant patients, equivalent to 0.3 patients per million per year.

NUTRITIONAL SUPPORT AND OVERALL MANAGEMENT

The main goals of management of CIPO are: (1) improvement of intestinal propulsion and (2) maintenance of adequate nutritional status including fluid and mineral balances. Indeed, as a consequence of chronic dysmotility, inadequate oral intake, increased losses (vomiting and diarrhea) and malabsorption, malnutrition can develop, and nutritional status should be systematically evaluated. If bacterial overgrowth is present, various treatment regimes are available, depending on the severity of the disease. Dietary education may be sufficient for patients with mild and moderate symptoms. If oral food intake becomes inadequate, nutritional support must be provided in the form of either enteral or parenteral nutrition.

Prokinetics

Whereas their effectiveness in terms of reducing clinical symptoms is poor, prokinetic drugs are systematically used in CIPO, probably because of their potential to improve digestive motility, as evidenced by manometric findings.[2–4] Lack of effectiveness is possibly explained by the poor intestinal bioavailability of oral drugs. In some cases, combinations of prokinetics could improve digestive motility.[5] New prokinetic drugs should be evaluated in the near future.

Treatment of Bacterial Overgrowth

Intestinal bacterial overgrowth has been well documented as a complication of intestinal motility disorders,[6,7] and it has been shown that promoting digestive motility reduces bacterial overgrowth.[2] Sequential antibiotic therapy is very effective in treating intestinal bacterial overgrowth and reducing malabsorption.[8] Correlations between bacterial translocation and an absence of migrating motor complex activity has been demonstrated and can result in a further impairment of the digestive motility disorder.[9] Systemic sepsis is a potentially life-threatening consequence of bacterial overgrowth.[10,11]

Dietary Measures

Dietary measures are influenced by disease phenotype and aim to provide sufficient intake of micro- and macronutrients orally.[12] Patients with gastroparesis usually feature diminished oral intake because of early satiety, whereas patients with predominantly small bowel involvement often suffer nausea, abdominal pain, and diarrhea. In individuals with delayed gastric emptying, liquid or blenderized food is better tolerated than solid food.[13] Oral intake should also be fractionated and divided into 5 to 6 meals per day. Dietary measures should also include the use of a low-lactose, low-fiber, low-fat diet to optimize gut motility and to decrease the risk of bacterial overgrowth and gastric bezoar formation. Associated multivitamin and micronutrient supplementation is also needed (iron, folate, calcium, and vitamins D, K, and B12) to prevent the development of specific deficiency states.[14]

Enteral Nutrition

Enteral feeding by ostomy is a potentially effective method of providing nutritional support, which could be used despite oral feeding intolerance. However, it should be commenced carefully with an iso-osmolar nutrient formulation delivered by slow continuous infusion rate to optimize tolerance and prevent enteral nutrition-related pneumonia. If this trial period is tolerated, the infusion rate and the volume of infusion can be increased progressively. An ostomy could be also helpful to provide venting.

Parenteral Nutrition

HPN is necessary in severe CIPO patients in whom there has been failure of other supportive methods.[15] Because of higher cost, morbidity and mortality, and the low probability of being able to wean off HPN, it should not be initiated before there has been an adequate trial of oral or enteral nutrition feeding.[14] Issues specific to the use of HPN in CIPO patients are relate to the impact of chronic bowel obstruction and poor oral intake.

- Higher fluid volume is required to prevent dehydration, especially in cases of refractory vomiting or permanent ostomy suction/drainage. Fluid volume requirements must also be adapted in real time because of frequent and variably fluctuating digestive losses (diarrhea, vomiting). The same is true for fluid and electrolyte balance and for sodium, potassium, and magnesium, in particular.
- More infusions occur per week (6–7 per week for CIPO patients versus 4–5 for short bowel syndrome; unpublished personal data).
- To prevent parenteral nutrition (PN)-related liver disease, especially in those maintained exclusively on HPN (ie, patients with intractable obstruction), lipid parenteral intake should be limited (to that minimal intake necessary to prevent fatty acid deficiency).
- Micronutrient and vitamin supplements (such as selenium, vitamins B1, B6, and E) should be provided and their intake adapted according to regular nutritional surveys.
- There is necessity to maintain minimal oral feeding to (1) reduce parenteral caloric needs and (2) prevent complications of being maintained exclusively on HPN (bacterial translocation, liver disease, biliary complications, intestinal partial villous atrophy, especially, that induced by bacterial overgrowth . . .)
- Mitochondrial cytopathies may require specific vitamin supplementation regimes: coenzyme Q10, ubiquinone or its synthetic variant, idébenone.[16]

Surgical Procedures

Surgical procedures often take place before or during CIPO management.[17–19] Surgery cannot be curative in this context, so its use should be limited to refractory form of CIPO and in very selected indications. The most common and effective surgical procedure is the creation of a venting or feeding ostomy.[20] Venting ostomies decrease the frequency of vomiting and of admission for acute obstructive symptoms and also prevent abdominal pain and retching in patients who have undergone antireflux surgery. Besides, gastrointestinal motility may improve as the bowel becomes less dilated.[1] Furthermore, a combined nasogastric-nasojejunal tube is available that allows simultaneous gastric suction and jejunal infusion.[21] Exploratory laparotomy could be done to lyse adhesions where there is a suspicion of mechanical bowel obstruction caused by a previous laparotomy. In those cases, full-thickness biopsy or limited small bowel resection can be performed to facilitate a detailed histopathologic study. Bowel resection or surgical bypass should be resisted at all cost. Only a very few patients with disease that is well documented to be isolated to a given segment can benefit from resection or bypass procedures.[22] On the contrary, those with extensive disease will not benefit and are likely to experience perioperative complications. In those rare cases in which patients with CIPO are nonresponsive to maximal medical and surgical therapy and have developed complications, such as dehydration or severe intestinal translocation, they may benefit from subtotal bowel resection[23–26] or intestinal transplantation.[12,27–29] Intestinal transplantation has become a life-saving procedure for patients with irreversible intestinal failure. The indications were defined as life-threatening complications of HPN, lack of venous access for HPN, chronic intestinal failure with a high risk of mortality, and primary disease-related poor quality of life despite optimal HPN. To date, approximately 1300 intestinal transplantations have been performed (40% in adult patients); approximately 8% of adults underwent transplantation for intestinal failure caused by CIPO.[28] Multivisceral transplantations were often performed for this indication with a 1-year patient and graft survival rates (approximately 80% and 65%, respectively) that were relatively similar to those for other etiologies of intestinal failure.[27] Intestinal transplantation should be considered in adult patients suffering from CIPO who have life-threatening complications related to PN.

Natural History

Pediatric forms of CIPO usually present at birth or in early infancy.[30,31] Adult forms occur in young people (20–40 years), with more women than men (sex ratio of 2:3) affected.[17–20] Symptoms of CIPO are directly related to ineffective propulsion and include the classic features of bowel obstruction, including nausea, vomiting, abdominal pain or distension, anorexia, and weight loss. Symptoms often are chronic and continuous and progressively increase in frequency and severity with time. There seems to be no difference in the nature of symptoms at the time of onset and at follow-up.[19] Sometimes CIPO is revealed only at the time of surgery for an acute obstructive episode mimicking mechanical bowel obstruction. In its more severe clinical form, CIPO manifests as total oral intolerance, permanent obstruction, intractable pain, and rapid loss of weight with protein energy malnutrition and life-threatening deficiencies, requiring HPN.

Long-term outcome is generally poor, despite surgical and medical therapy. Three types of complications are frequently reported in CIPO: (1) HPN-related complications (catheter related sepsis, thrombosis, PN-related liver disease)[32]; (2) complications related to associated diseases, such as renal and urinary, cardiac, and central and peripheral nervous system diseases; and (3) specific complications of CIPO (dehydration, metabolic disturbances, bacterial translocation, peritonitis, gastroesophageal reflux disease with or without Barrett's mucosa, aspiration pneumonia).[33] In the literature, the incidence of PN-related complications does not seem to differ between CIPO-related and other causes of intestinal failure. However, one would predict that PN-related liver disease may develop more rapidly in patients with CIPO because of the presence of bacterial overgrowth and the occurrence of bacterial translocation.

In CIPO, HPN is required from 60% to 80% of infants and 20% to 50% of adults.[17–19,30,34] In infants, long-term outcome is characterized by a 10% to 25% likelihood of mortality before reaching adulthood. Although part of the morbidity and mortality is attributable to complications of treatment, including surgery and parenteral nutrition, studies have identified some factors predictive of a poor outcome in children: short small bowel, exclusively parenteral nutrition with enteral feeding not possible, urinary tract involvement, neonatal forms of CIPO, absence of migrating motor complex activity on manometry, and the presence of a visceral myopathy.[30,31] Congenital CIPO has also been associated with increased morbidity and mortality compared with acquired forms.[35] While initial reports revealed a 25% to 30% mortality rate at early follow-up,[17,31] recently, 2 studies reported a 10% mortality rate after a mean follow-up of, respectively, 17.5 and 4.6 years.[18,19]

In Our Practice

In adults, the clinical course, long-term outcome, and prognostic factors are less well known because available data are limited to clinical series reporting on small numbers of patients of heterogeneous etiology and variable disease severity. From January 1980 to April 2006, we reviewed the medical records of all consecutive adult patients with a diagnosis of CIPO followed up at our institution for HPN.[36] In this population (51 CIPO patients), from the first symptom occurrence to the time of diagnosis, a body mass index (BMI) decrease from 20 ± 3.4 kg/m^2 to 17 ± 3.2 kg/m^2 was observed. Delay between first symptom occurrence and HPN initiation was 3.2 (range, 0–23) years. HPN duration was 2.5 (range, 0–21) years. The number of infusions per week was 5.9 ± 1.4, with a volume per infusion of 2354 ± 793 mL and a total energy input of 1444 ± 349 kcal per infusion. The degree of HPN dependence was 64% ± 25%. A clinically important improvement in BMI from 16.8 ± 3.2 kg/m^2 to 18.5 ± 2.5 kg/m^2 was observed with dietary and HPN management, although reversal to premorbid BMI was not achieved. Considering the oral intake, 33% had adaptive hyperphagia, whereas 30% had a total oral intolerance to oral intake. At the end of follow-up, the Buzby index was 82% ± 10% and, of the 51 patients, 33% and 55% still featured moderate and severe malnutrition, respectively.

Surgery was required in 84% of cases with 3.0 ± 3.3 procedures per patient. Nineteen patients (37%) had undergone surgery at the time of their first presentation and before the diagnosis of CIPO. After the diagnosis of CIPO, a clinically significant reduction in the mean (per patient per year) number of surgical procedures was observed, decreasing from 2.2 ± 5.3 to 0.3 ± 0.5, and, specifically, the number of exploratory laparotomies decreased from 0.57 ± 1.4 to 0.008 ± 0.02. Surgical procedures were explorative laparotomy in 43% of cases, intestinal resection in 67%, and venting or end ostomy in 69%. Intestinal resections included subtotal colectomy (n = 14), small bowel resection (n = 19), ileocolonic resection (n = 13), and subtotal small bowel resection (n = 8). Twenty-eight venting (or feeding) gastrostomies were performed during follow-up.

Survival of CIPO patients was not significantly different than that in our population of short bowel patients (n = 309; 78% vs 72% at 5 years, P = .07). In multivariate analysis, mortality was significantly decreased when there was an ability to restore oral feeding at baseline (hazard ratio [HR], 0.2 [0.06–0.65]; P = .008) and where symptoms occurred before the age of 20 (HR, 0.18 [0.04–0.88]; P = .03). In contrast, mortality was significantly increased in systemic sclerosis (HR, 10.4 [1.6–67.9]; P = .01).

Thirty-nine (76.5%) patients were permanently dependent on HPN. Six patients had experienced intermittent periods of weaning off HPN. Three of these 6 patients were definitively weaned off after a mean HPN period of 7 (range, 3–16) months. The other 3 patients restarted HPN after a mean delay of 70 (range, 31–130) months. Actuarial HPN dependence probabilities were 94%, 75%, and 72% at 1, 2, and 5 years, respectively. The likelihood of weaning off HPN was significantly lower in the idiopathic form of CIPO (HR, 30.4, confidence interval (CI) [2–489]; $P = .02$) and where the postabsorptive plasma citrulline level was lower than 20 μmol/L (HR, 17.3, CI [1–292]; $P = .05$).

SUMMARY

The management of CIPO remains difficult and requires a multidisciplinary approach. In adult patients with CIPO on HPN, the 10-year survival rate was 68%. Long-term HPN dependence does not seem to be associated with a significant increase in mortality and morbidity. HPN could be a safe and efficient approach to the management of intestinal failure caused by CIPO, with restoring oral intake and lowering hospitalization frequency as major goals of treatment.

REFERENCES

1. Di Lorenzo C. Pseudo-obstruction: current approaches. Gastroenterology 1999;116(4):980–7.
2. Soudah HC, Hasler WL, Owyang C, et al. Effect of octreotide on intestinal motility and bacterial overgrowth in scleroderma. N Engl J Med 1991;325(21):1461–7.
3. Tack J, Janssens J, Vantrappen G, et al. Effect of erythromycin on gastric motility in controls and in diabetic gastroparesis. Gastroenterology 1992;103(1):72–9.
4. Quigley EM. Chronic intestinal pseudo-obstruction. Curr Treat Options Gastroenterol 1999;2(3):239–50.
5. Verne GN, Eaker EY, Hardy E, et al. Effect of octreotide and erythromycin on idiopathic and scleroderma-associated intestinal pseudoobstruction. Dig Dis Sci 1995;40(9):1892–901.
6. Riordan SM, McIver CJ, Walker BM, et al. Bacteriological method for detecting small intestinal hypomotility. Am J Gastroenterol 1996;91(11):2399–405.
7. Parson AJ, Brzechwa-Ajdukiewicz A, McCarthy CF, et al. Intestinal pseudo-obstruction with bacterial overgrowth in the small intestine. Am J Dig Dis 1969;14(3):200–5.
8. Attar A, Flourie B, Rambaud JC, et al. Antibiotic efficacy in small intestinal bacterial overgrowth-related chronic diarrhea: a crossover, randomized trial. Gastroenterology 1999;117(4):794–7.
9. Nieuwenhuijs VB, Verheem, van Duijvenbode-Beumer H, et al. The role of interdigestive small bowel motility in the regulation of gut microflora, bacterial overgrowth, and bacterial translocation in rats. Ann Surg 1998;228(2):188–93.
10. Berg RD. Bacterial translocation from the gastrointestinal tract. Adv Exp Med Biol 1999;473:11–30.
11. Madl C, Druml W, et al. Gastrointestinal disorders of the critically ill. Systemic consequences of ileus. Best Pract Res Clin Gastroenterol 2003;17(3):445–56.
12. Scolapio JS, Ukleja A, Bouras EP, et al. Nutritional management of chronic intestinal pseudo-obstruction. J Clin Gastroenterol 1999;28(4):306–12.
13. Camilleri M, Phillips SF. Acute and chronic intestinal pseudo-obstruction. Adv Intern Med 1991;36:287–306.
14. Smith DS, Williams CS, Ferris CD, et al. Diagnosis and treatment of chronic gastroparesis and chronic intestinal pseudo-obstruction. Gastroenterol Clin North Am 2003;32(2):619–58.
15. Messing B, Joly F. Guidelines for management of home parenteral adult chronic intestinal failure patients. Gastroenterology 2006;130(2):S43–51.

16. Geromel V, Darin N, Chrétien D, et al. Coenzyme Q(10) and idebenone in the therapy of respiratory chain diseases: rationale and comparative benefits. Mol Genet Metab 2002;77(1–2):21–30.
17. Hanks JB, Weber WB. Chronic primary intestinal pseudo-obstruction. Surgery 1981; 89(2):175–82.
18. Mann SD, Debinski HS, Kamm MA, et al. Clinical characteristics of chronic idiopathic intestinal pseudo-obstruction in adults. Gut 1997;41(5):675–81.
19. Stanghellini V, Cogliandro RF, De Giorgio R, et al. Natural history of chronic idiopathic intestinal pseudo-obstruction in adults: a single center study. Clin Gastroenterol Hepatol 2005;3(5):449–58.
20. Pitt HA, Mann LL, Berquist WE, et al. Chronic intestinal pseudo-obstruction. Management with total parenteral nutrition and a venting enterostomy. Arch Surg 1985; 120(5):614–8.
21. Patrick PG, Marulendra S, Kirby DF, et al. Endoscopic nasogastric-jejunal feeding tube placement in critically ill patients. Gastrointest Endosc 1997;45(1):72–6.
22. Murr MM, Sarr MG, Camilleri M, et al. The surgeon's role in the treatment of chronic intestinal pseudoobstruction. Am J Gastroenterol 1995;90(12):2147–51.
23. Schuffler MD, Leon SH, Krishnamurthy S, et al. Intestinal pseudoobstruction caused by a new form of visceral neuropathy: palliation by radical small bowel resection. Gastroenterology 1985; 89(5):1152–6.
24. Mughal MM, Irving MH. Treatment of end stage chronic intestinal pseudo-obstruction by subtotal enterectomy and home parenteral nutrition. Gut 1988;29(11):1613–7.
25. Joly F, Zeballos J, Benoist S, et al. Subtotal small bowel resection (SBR) in chronic intestinal pseudo-obstruction (CIPO) refractory to treatment. Clin Nutr 2003;22(S1): S56–7.
26. Buchman AL, Scolapio J, Fryer J, et al. AGA technical review on short bowel syndrome and intestinal transplantation. Gastroenterology 2003;124(4):1111–34.
27. Masetti M, Di Benedetto F, Cautero N, et al. Intestinal transplantation for chronic intestinal pseudo-obstruction in adult patients. Am J Transplant 2004;4(5):826–9.
28. Grant D, Abu-Elmagd K, Reyes J, et al. 2003 report of the intestine transplant registry: a new era has dawned. Ann Surg 2005;241(4): 607–13.
29. Blondon H, Polivka M, Joly F, et al. Digestive smooth muscle mitochondrial myopathy in patients with mitochondrial-neuro-gastro-intestinal encephalomyopthy (MNGIE). Gastroenterol Clin Biol 2005;29:773–8.
30. Faure C, Goulet O, Ategbo S, et al. Chronic intestinal pseudoobstruction syndrome: clinical analysis, outcome, and prognosis in 105 children. French-Speaking Group of Pediatric Gastroenterology. Dig Dis Sci 1999;44(5):953–9.
31. Vargas JH, Sachs P, Ament ME, et al. Chronic intestinal pseudo-obstruction syndrome in pediatrics: results of a national survey by members of the North American Society of Gastroenterology and Nutrition. J Pediatr Gastroenterol Nutr 1988;7(3):323–32.
32. Howard L, Ashley C. Management of complications in patients receiving home parenteral nutrition. Gastroenterology 2003;124(6):1651–61.
33. Joly F, Amiot A, Coffin B, et al. Chronic intestinal pseudo-obstruction. Gastroenterol Clin Biol 2006;30:975–85.
34. Mousa H, Hyman PE, Cocjin J, et al. Long-term outcome of congenital intestinal pseudoobstruction. Dig Dis Sci 2002;47(10):2298–305.
35. Huang YC, Lee HC, Huang FY, et al. Neonatal onset chronic intestinal pseudo-obstruction syndrome. Clin Pediatr (Phila) 1995;34(5):241–7.
36. Amiot A, Joly F, Alves A, et al. Long-term outcome of chronic intestinal pseudo-obstruction adult patients requiring home parenteral nutrition. Am J Gastroenterol 2009;104(5):1262–70.

Index

Note: Page numbers of article titles are in **bold face** type.

Gastroenterol Clin N Am 40 (2011) 853–863
doi:10.1016/S0889-8553(11)00098-7

J

L

M

United States Postal Service

Statement of Ownership, Management, and Circulation
(All Periodicals Publications Except Requestor Publications)

1. Publication Title: Gastroenterology Clinics of North America
2. Publication Number: 0 0 0 - 2 7 9
3. Filing Date: 9/16/11
4. Issue Frequency: Mar, Jun, Sep, Dec
5. Number of Issues Published Annually: 4
6. Annual Subscription Price: $282.00
7. Complete Mailing Address of Known Office of Publication (*Not printer*) (*Street, city, county, state, and ZIP+4®*)

Elsevier Inc.
360 Park Avenue South
New York, NY 10010-1710

Contact Person: Amy S. Beacham
Telephone (Include area code): 215-239-3687

8. Complete Mailing Address of Headquarters or General Business Office of Publisher (*Not printer*)

Elsevier Inc., 360 Park Avenue South, New York, NY 10010-1710

9. Full Names and Complete Mailing Addresses of Publisher, Editor, and Managing Editor (*Do not leave blank*)

Publisher (*Name and complete mailing address*)

Kim Murphy, Elsevier, Inc., 1600 John F. Kennedy Blvd. Suite 1800, Philadelphia, PA 19103-2899

Editor (*Name and complete mailing address*)

Kerry Holland, Elsevier, Inc., 1600 John F. Kennedy Blvd. Suite 1800, Philadelphia, PA 19103-2899

Managing Editor (*Name and complete mailing address*)

Sarah Barth, Elsevier, Inc., 1600 John F. Kennedy Blvd. Suite 1800, Philadelphia, PA 19103-2899

10. Owner (*Do not leave blank. If the publication is owned by a corporation, give the name and address of the corporation immediately followed by the names and addresses of all stockholders owning or holding 1 percent or more of the total amount of stock. If not owned by a corporation, give the names and addresses of the individual owners. If owned by a partnership or other unincorporated firm, give its name and address as well as those of each individual owner. If the publication is published by a nonprofit organization, give its name and address.*)

Full Name	Complete Mailing Address
Wholly owned subsidiary of	4520 East-West Highway
Reed/Elsevier, US holdings	Bethesda, MD 20814

11. Known Bondholders, Mortgagees, and Other Security Holders Owning or Holding 1 Percent or More of Total Amount of Bonds, Mortgages, or Other Securities. If none, check box ☐ None

Full Name	Complete Mailing Address
N/A	

12. Tax Status (*For completion by nonprofit organizations authorized to mail at nonprofit rates*) (*Check one*)
The purpose, function, and nonprofit status of this organization and the exempt status for federal income tax purposes:
☐ Has Not Changed During Preceding 12 Months
☐ Has Changed During Preceding 12 Months (*Publisher must submit explanation of change with this statement*)

PS Form 3526, September 2007 (Page 1 of 3 (Instructions Page 3)) PSN 7530-01-000-9931 **PRIVACY NOTICE**: See our Privacy policy in www.usps.com

13. Publication Title: Gastroenterology Clinics of North America
14. Issue Date for Circulation Data Below: September 2011

15. Extent and Nature of Circulation			Average No. Copies Each Issue During Preceding 12 Months	No. Copies of Single Issue Published Nearest to Filing Date
a. Total Number of Copies (*Net press run*)			1449	1100
b. Paid Circulation (By Mail and Outside the Mail)	(1)	Mailed Outside-County Paid Subscriptions Stated on PS Form 3541. (*Include paid distribution above nominal rate, advertiser's proof copies, and exchange copies*)	528	458
	(2)	Mailed In-County Paid Subscriptions Stated on PS Form 3541 (*Include paid distribution above nominal rate, advertiser's proof copies, and exchange copies*)		
	(3)	Paid Distribution Outside the Mails Including Sales Through Dealers and Carriers, Street Vendors, Counter Sales, and Other Paid Distribution Outside USPS®	366	355
	(4)	Paid Distribution by Other Classes Mailed Through the USPS (e.g. First-Class Mail®)		
c. Total Paid Distribution (*Sum of 15b (1), (2), (3), and (4)*)			894	813
d. Free or Nominal Rate Distribution (By Mail and Outside the Mail)	(1)	Free or Nominal Rate Outside-County Copies Included on PS Form 3541	95	88
	(2)	Free or Nominal Rate In-County Copies Included on PS Form 3541		
	(3)	Free or Nominal Rate Copies Mailed at Other Classes Through the USPS (e.g. First-Class Mail)		
	(4)	Free or Nominal Rate Distribution Outside the Mail (Carriers or other means)		
e. Total Free or Nominal Rate Distribution (Sum of 15d (1), (2), (3) and (4)			95	88
f. Total Distribution (Sum of 15c and 15e)			989	901
g. Copies not Distributed (See instructions to publishers #4 (page #3))			460	199
h. Total (Sum of 15f and g)			1449	1100
i. Percent Paid (15c divided by 15f times 100)			90.39%	90.23%

16. Publication of Statement of Ownership
☐ If the publication is a general publication, publication of this statement is required. Will be printed in the **December 2011** issue of this publication. ☐ Publication not required

17. Signature and Title of Editor, Publisher, Business Manager, or Owner

Amy S. Beacham – Senior Inventory Distribution Coordinator

Date: September 16, 2011

I certify that all information furnished on this form is true and complete. I understand that anyone who furnishes false or misleading information on this form or who omits material or information requested on the form may be subject to criminal sanctions (including fines and imprisonment) and/or civil sanctions (including civil penalties).

PS Form 3526, September 2007 (Page 2 of 3)

Printed and bound by CPI Group (UK) Ltd, Croydon, CR0 4YY
03/10/2024
01040449-0015